The Birds,
the Bees,
and the
Elephant
in the Room

The Birds, the Bees, and the Elephant

TALKING TO YOUR KIDS ABOUT SEX AND OTHER SENSITIVE TOPICS

and the

Elephant

RACHEL COLER MULHOLLAND MS, LPC

in the Room

UNION
SQUARE
& CO.

NEW YORK

UNION SQUARE & CO. and the distinctive Union Square & Co. logo
are trademarks of Sterling Publishing Co., Inc.

Union Square & Co., LLC, is a subsidiary of Sterling Publishing Co., Inc.

This publication is intended for informational purposes only. The publisher does not claim that this publication shall provide or guarantee any benefits, healing, cure, or any results in any respect. This publication is not intended to provide or replace medical advice, treatment, or diagnosis or be a substitute to consulting with a physician or other licensed medical or health-care providers. The publisher and author shall not be liable or responsible for any use or application of any content contained in this publication or any adverse effects, consequence, loss, or damage of any type resulting or arising from, directly or indirectly, the use or application of any content contained in this publication.

The author and editor have made every effort to reproduce the substance of the conversations relied on in this book but some have been edited and condensed for clarity and space. Names and identifying details have been changed at the individuals' request and/or to preserve the author's obligation to uphold patient confidentiality.

ISBN 978-1-4549-5370-8
ISBN 978-1-4549-5371-5 (e-book)

For information about custom editions, special sales, and premium purchases,
please contact specialsales@unionsquareandco.com.

Printed in Canada

2 4 6 8 10 9 7 5 3 1

unionsquareandco.com

Interior design: Christine A. Heun
Cover design: Jennifer Heuer

Cover Images: Getty Images: Antagain/E+ (Bee);
Nicholas Brink/500px (Elephant); Shutterstock.com: Svetlana Foote (Bird)

For J.W.A.V.—I love you too much

Contents

Introduction:
What to Expect in This Book

"Sooooo here's a story from A to Z, you wanna get with me . . ."

Man, it's kinda hot.

These shorts are itchy.

Wonder what Dad wants . . .

I wonder if I can go to the pool this afternoon . . .

My eleven-year-old mind was going through its usual chatter one afternoon in July 1997 when my dad sat me down on the front steps of our small-town Minnesota home. I remember it distinctly: the heat of the concrete steps, the buzz of the cicadas. I remember my dad's kind face, and how I could smell summertime and Old Spice as I sat next to him. I even remember that he was wearing a red T-shirt with the sleeves cut off, most likely because he was planning to do some work in the garage after he took care of this piece of business. I remember thinking, *Remember when Mom fell down these steps and cut her arm to the bone? And decided to give us an anatomy lesson before heading to the ER?* (True story—it's on page 66.)

I'm not certain how my parents came to the conclusion that my dad needed to have The Talk with me that afternoon—it's not like they'd been stingy with scientific information during my childhood. They had always held the belief that if a child was old enough to ask the question, they were old enough to be given an answer, and scientific resources were abundant at my house (as you'll discover on page 35). But for whatever reason, there I was, waiting and wondering what my dad wanted to talk to me about.

It's funny to me that I remember this particular moment, because I actually have very few distinct memories of childhood—one of the frustrating bugs of being a human with attention deficit hyperactivity disorder (ADHD).

Anyway, you know that moment in a movie where the protagonist just got a momentous piece of life-changing news, and instead of continuing to hear the information they're receiving, the audio cuts to their inner monologue? As if their brain has kicked up the volume on the voice in their head as a defense mechanism so they don't have to hear anything else? You follow? Okay, that EXACT THING happened to me when it became clear what my dad was trying to talk to me about. When he decided it was time to make sure he could check "sex ed" off the Parenting To-Do List, my brain stepped in, and instead of hearing anything he was trying to tell me, it said, "ABSOLUTELY NOT. YOU ARE GOING TO SING THE ENTIRE SPICE GIRLS ALBUM IN YOUR HEAD INSTEAD."

So I guess Adult Me can thank my dad and my tendency for escapism for my flawless bar karaoke execution of "Wannabe," but when it comes to my understanding of all the ins and outs of sex (pardon the euphemism), I can't exactly thank The Talk.

I approached my own parenting journey with that memory firmly at the forefront of my mind. I knew that I entered adulthood with *much* more information than many of my peers, and yet I still felt flat-footed about a lot of things. Clearly having The Talk wasn't an effective method for my young brain, so how *had* I gotten the information I did? How did I know about sperm and egg, about the forty-week gestation period, about how people in relationships should treat each other? And how could I improve upon the foundation my parents gave me? How could I help my own children feel empowered and generally safe (both feelings I had as a young adult) while also helping them avoid some of the pitfalls I experienced in my early sexual years?

It was in attempting to answer these questions for myself that I decided to approach "the birds and the bees" the way I have—a firm set of requirements for my foundations and delineating the conversations into "mechanics" and "specifics." This strategy worked well for me as my kids were growing, and in the spring of 2021, on a whim, I decided to share the result of a "mechanics" conversation on TikTok. In a 60-second video, my then six-year-old (whom I call Turkey on social media to protect her privacy) described menstruation to me. With my daughter off camera, I asked, "What happens every month in a uterus?"

"It says 'I'm going to have a baby . . . I'm going to DECORATE!" she replied enthusiastically.

"'I'm gonna decorate,' and how does it do that?"

"It decorates itself and puts some tissues on, like blood!"

"Tissues on the walls, mm-hmm! And are they nutrient-rich? Are they the perfect place for a baby to grow?" I asked. Off camera, she nodded sagely.

This kid loves to share knowledge, so I encouraged some follow-up: "And then what happens?"

"And then when it finds out we're not, it says 'UGH, FINE,'" she says with *all* the attitude, "and it RIPS IT ALL DOWN!"

"And it comes out as . . . ?"

"Blood," she answers, matter-of-factly.

"And what happens if a baby goes in there? It . . . ?"

"GROWS!"

"It grows!" I proudly confirm.

I put her to bed, added some captions to the video, and posted it to my fledgling TikTok page. I had less than a hundred followers and didn't expect the video to go to anyone other than the friends and family who had given me pity follows when I started my page. It was my fourth or fifth video, and the ones I'd posted previously had gotten a couple hundred views at most.

In the next 24 hours, that video demonstrating how to unabashedly and unashamedly address the elephant in the room amassed over *one million views*.

Not only did it amass views, it amassed comments—people were blown away by Turkey's knowledge. Some folks were against her knowing about her own body—commenting things like "Why does this baby know this stuff? Who would do that?" But the majority of people were curious about how she had developed that level of understanding, and asked questions about what else she knew or how they could help their kids develop the same education and autonomy. Over the next several months, I continued to create and post content—sometimes about body talk, sometimes parenting, and sometimes just moments with my kids or fun trends.

A few things have become clear as my page has grown. First, parents are still feeling confused about and intimidated by how to approach talking about sex and bodies with their kids. Second, parents and nonparents alike are actively seeking information on how to prepare themselves for these conversations. And third, they are doing this because they feel their own education in the subject was not what it could have been.

The following stories, chapters, and sample scripts are my attempt to meet this need in a tangible, easy-to-reference way. The book is organized in a chronological but also stand-alone way, meaning that you can read it front to back, but also use it for in-the-moment reference. The first chapters of the book are Foundations—pieces that are necessary in order to have successful conversations with your kids at all ages. Foundations are meant to address the Trust Conundrum—or, as my sister puts it, "If I can't ask you about my penis when I'm young, I can't ask you about where to put it when I'm older." Foundations also address both the overarching concept of Consent and what I call Consent for Knowledge—which means recognizing that body talk and sex education need to be conversations, not lectures. Kids need to know about their bodies and about sex, but they also deserve to only know what they're *ready* to know. The middle chapters are what I've deemed Mechanics—the earliest conversations you'll have with your kids about How It All Works. These are the nuts and bolts (again with the euphemisms!) of how bodies function—from self-exploration to periods to the dreaded "where do babies come from?" The final chapters are Specifics—the conversations we have as children grow up, realizing the interpersonal aspects of our bodies and the human experience. This section dives further into consent and how we navigate budding romantic relationships and new feelings of attraction to others, and, probably most importantly, how to keep yourself safe as you wade into the wider world. These conversations can be some of the most difficult to have, but (as we know) they're the most critical for giving children their best chances at being happy, protecting their health, and staying safe.

Each chapter includes not only information for you as a parent, but also at least one sample script that you can use to help plan out how to talk with your child. The scripts generally utilize the same inclusive language that the rest of the text uses, and acknowledge trans and nonbinary identities as valid and important. Through this text, unless it's specified otherwise, "men" means *all* men, and "women" means *all* women. And while no conversation with your child is going to exactly mirror the scripts in the book, the general ideas are likely to be similar.

This book is designed as a guide for you as a parent, but also as a road map for you and your kids to use together. Sometimes even the best parent-child relationships arrive at a point where one party (or both!) feels like they just can't say/ask/express what they need to. In those moments, I hope you feel confident reaching for this book. Though a lot of us find ourselves dreading these talks, I hope this book can help you find the humor, relax in the humanity, and ultimately enjoy the comfort of knowing you've armed your kids with information—something that can never be taken away from them.

PART 1

FOUNDATIONS

I know it's tempting to jump ahead to the chapters that you think might answer all you and your children's pressing questions, but I want you to Pump. The. Brakes. I want you to know that I'm proud of you for starting at the beginning, and if you're someone who is coming back here to read after having skipped ahead, it's okay—I'm proud of you, too. It's possible you picked up this book well in advance of your kiddo asking you anything you're not sure how to answer, but it's equally possible that you grabbed this book off the shelf in hopes that it can help you tackle something your kid asked you at bedtime just last night.

You have to remember that in most forms of parenting, we're playing the long game. We're investing in little things now that turn into much bigger things later. That's what this first section is about—the small daily foundational values that we instill in our relationships with our children that shape how the Big Things happen later. Think of it like watching Bob Ross create a masterpiece on *The Joy of Painting*. He starts with a canvas prepped with Liquid White and then he builds. With thoughtful, well-planned layers, considerate brushstrokes, and a few "happy accidents," he manages to create something amazing. The same thing applies to the Foundations contained in this book.

The Foundation of Unconditional Positive Regard asks us to consider how our words and actions convey our feelings to our child daily—especially when things get difficult. The Foundation of Curiosity encourages us as parents to foster a sense of curiosity about life—from small daily interactions to the big mysteries of the universe—to increase our children's sense of safety in asking questions. And the Foundations of Consent and Consent for Knowledge provide us guidance on how to raise children who feel confident setting and respecting boundaries for their minds, bodies, and hearts.

Altogether, this section asks you to reflect on how you relate to each Foundation both with your children and in the rest of your life. All the information you will read going forward is made more useful and personalized by having reflected on your own core values and how they interact with the Foundations here. You get to decide how you can be truthful, factual, supportive, and comfortable discussing complex topics within the framework of your own morals, values, and communication style, and always reminding your child that at the end of the day, you'll be there for them. As you'll soon read, "I will always love you" sounds simple, and it is . . . but it also isn't.

CHAPTER 1

Unconditional Positive Regard

"I KNOOOOOOW," my daughter groans in the kind of exasperated sigh only an eight-year-old can muster (the groans and sighs I get from my sixteen- and five-year-olds are distinctly different). "There's nothing I can do to make you stop loving me, I KNOW . . . But what if I MURDER SOMEONE?"

"Well, I'll definitely need to know WHY you murdered them—maybe it was necessary! But I'll still love you." I answered.

"What if I murder SANTA?!"

"Did he come down the chimney and you thought he was a robber? Or was it just like . . . because you could? Regardless, I'll still love you. I just need to plan whether I'm visiting you in prison or learning about stand-your-ground law."

It's at this point that I've completely lost the plot with this kid, and she's gotten exactly what she wanted—confirmation that I'll never stop loving her, and attention in the form of an absolutely ludicrous conversation.

This particular example of unconditional positive regard is emblematic of how conversations with my kids regarding my feelings for them typically go. First, I remind them at some perfectly mundane time that there's nothing they can do to get me to stop loving them. Then they roll their eyes at having to hear this exact phrase for the 50/100/1,000th time and follow up their giant sigh with some highly unlikely scenario to test the theory. We banter back and forth a bit about exactly how this ridiculous turn of events might have come to pass, but ultimately, they land right back where they started—with a mother who will never, not *ever*, stop loving them. Regardless of what they do, regardless of who they love, regardless of the bad choices they might make or questions they might feel uncomfortable asking me—there is nothing in the whole wide world that will make me stop loving them.

The concept of unconditional positive regard was made popular by humanistic psychologist Carl Rogers in the 1950s. Though the idea is generally used in psychology to describe the way a clinician should treat their client—providing unconditional support by recognizing their innate ability to grow and change—it's easy to apply to caregivers and their children. Think of it this way: You, as their primary, most loving grown-up, can see both the tiny child before you and the awesomely cool grown-up they're going to be . . . at the same time. That feeling—knowing your child is an unbelievably amazing future grown-up—is the beginning of unconditional positive regard.

Unconditional positive regard is *not* the same as unconditional love, which is the bare minimum. It's the idea that in addition to loving your child, you also respect your child and their personhood. You recognize that they are a whole person, separate from you, who deserves your care, attention, and esteem. It does not mean that you have no boundaries for your child; it does not mean that you cannot help your child learn morality; it is not unconditional "yes" or "they'll grow out of it" without guidance. It means specifically that you love your child enough to provide them with the safest and healthiest way to grow up that you can.

I believe that the unconditional positive regard of a primary caregiver is the first, most important foundational understanding to foster in children. This is rooted in both my experience as a parent, and also as a counselor. As a trained mental health practitioner, I've worked with children from early childhood all the way into early adulthood, and one of the most common themes I've recognized is that many children felt the most comfortable talking about hard things and asking me difficult questions when they feel sure I wouldn't be mad at them for talking or asking. I came to the conclusion that children acted this way in part because they viewed question asking the same way they viewed any other behavior—as something that would result in a response somewhere on the spectrum between praise and punishment—and asking a "bad" question the same way they viewed making a mistake. And for many of these kids, mistakes meant shame and punishment. To me, the connection was clear: The best way for me to help my children feel comfortable and confident asking me the hard questions was to show them that asking would never be a mistake—and that mistakes don't always mean punishment. Research shows that recognition for positive behavior not only helps reinforce positive behavior, it also aids in identity development, moral reasoning, and social thinking. So our job, then, as parents or caregivers, is to encourage the behavior we most want to see: open communication, trust, and, when the going gets tough, what my kids and I call "going toward love." This encouragement starts by figuring out how to *prove* to our kids that we are worthy. We start by *expressing* our unconditional love and *showing* them our unconditional positive regard.

You might be thinking expressing unconditional love is achieved with a sentiment like "I love you to the moon and back" or "I love you more than the universe" or any of the myriad of expressions of great love. But we know that children, especially young children, tend to be much more literal than those phrases account for. While we, as adults, have the abstract thinking necessary to understand that these expressions are meant to be interpreted as boundless love, kids don't understand them that way until they, too, have developed the ability for abstract thought (usually as they enter adolescence). That's why the phrase we use in our house—"there's nothing you can do to make me stop loving you"—is said the way it is. It is an explicit, unarguable, definable, and finite expression of the truth: that there is no question, thought, or action that my kids can have or do that will change my feelings for them.

As I mentioned, the way I choose to present information to children is primarily based on their cognitive development. Scientists have been interested in cognitive development—the way people learn to think—for a long time, and several theories have been proposed to explain how kids' brains grow and change over time. One of these, Jean Piaget's widely known theory of cognitive development, is the basis for many approaches and interventions for children, including the suggestions in this book. This theory states that cognitive development occurs over the course of the entire life span, and it can be broken into distinct stages.

The first stage of cognitive development, from birth to roughly age two, is called the sensorimotor stage. This is the time in a child's life when they are learning the most by interacting physically with the world around them. It's the stage of putting everything in their mouths and grabbing fistfuls of anything nearby—including your hair and their own bodies.

The next stage is the preoperational stage of development, from right about when they turn three until roughly age seven. Kids in this stage have usually learned to communicate and have the ability to express themselves, but they have a lot of difficulty understanding other people's points of view. They struggle to recognize that people may have different feelings about a situation than they do and have to have questions answered in a way that correlates to something they already know. As they grow through this period, kids learn to understand basic concepts like simple cause and effect, and love to know "why." They may even endeavor to answer their own questions with magical thinking instead of seeking out actual answers.

As kids gain the ability to see other perspectives and engage with ideas using logic, they enter what is called the concrete operational stage. Kids in this stage still love to know the answers to questions, but they can begin to look at evidence and come to conclusions based on the information in front of them. Kids are typically in the concrete operational stage from the age of seven until the age of eleven. While kids this age begin to demonstrate a more adult-like engagement with information, they still struggle to consider abstract or hypothetical ideas and scenarios. They do best when information can be related to a concrete example or demonstration that is familiar to them.

The stage of development that carries children into adult life is called the formal operational stage. Children (and adults) who have developed into this stage are able to mentally manipulate information presented to them and apply several modes of thinking to solve problems and find answers to their questions. At roughly age twelve, kids start engaging with hypothetical thought. They are able to consider the influence of several variables at a time, multiple outcomes, and how their thoughts and actions may influence those outcomes. Kids this age also begin to demonstrate metacognition, or "thinking about thinking"—they can gain introspection and see how their thoughts influence their own feelings, choices, and behaviors.

"There's nothing you can do to make me stop loving you" became my family's go-to phrase because it is easily understood starting from the moment they recognize that I have my own thoughts and feelings (right around age four). Now, I'll grant you—the phrase *is* a bit cumbersome. It can be a mouthful even at the best of times, so it's not the *only* expression of great love we use in our house. "I love you infinity and beyond" is tossed around with ease—so much so that I have it tattooed on my arm in my late husband's handwriting. My eldest child understands that infinity is limitless, and my youngest children will eventually understand the abstract idea of a number that never ends—so we will keep using the expression. We also indulge in finding things we love each other "more than": "I love you more than Indian food," "I love you more than dance," "I love you more than video games," "I love you more than this house and money and our car and everything I own." Depending on the seriousness of the mood, we can range from loving each other more than something barely tolerated—"I love you more than TOENAIL CHIP COOKIES"—to something sacred: "I love you more than my Grandpa Bear." This phrase is almost miraculous in its utility—I can use it to defuse a tense situation, dry tears, bring giggles, and infuse even a mundane moment with love.

I also love to ambush my children with "I love you." The game is easy enough in the beginning—the aim is to truly surprise them with an unexpected "I love you." When the kids are little, it's cake to win, because they never see it coming:

"Guess what?"

"What?!"

"I LOVE YOU!"

It quickly—around age four or five—starts to earn you a groan and an "I *know*." But shortly thereafter the kids start trying to beat you at your own game. "Guess what?" "You love me." Then you get to pick your reaction:

"I mean, DUH, but also—you have a booger on your nose."

Or: "Oh, gross. Thanks."

OR you can choose to reply:

"HOW DID YOU KNOW?!"

This response is my favorite, because it allows me to check in on the ways my child feels the most loved. Often they'll report that they know I love them because I tell them all the time. But sometimes they'll say "because you cuddle me" or "because you come to my recitals" or "because you are kind to my friends." I can take mental stock of the ways my child feels the most seen and supported, and make sure I'm continuing the behaviors that help them feel loved.

Even if we're cycling through all these expressions of great love on a daily basis, it bears repeating that they will not replace "There's nothing you can do to make me stop loving you." And that's because the goal of the phrase is simple: to cultivate a sense of both safety and security in my children. I want them to know that while I may express negative emotions ("I'm sorry, you spilled *what* on my bed?") or dole out natural consequences for choices that were ill-made ("You snuck extra computer time and made all of us late for the day because you couldn't get out of bed, so the router is on lockdown starting at nine p.m. to help you develop a better rhythm"), the outcomes of their mistakes will never be "You are nothing to me. I don't have a child with your name."

That being said, the sense of safety and security that children feel is influenced *far* more by actions than promises. We want them to know that not only do we love them unconditionally, we also respect them as individuals. Our children are learning How to People, and they are going to make a *lot* of mistakes and missteps in the process. They are going to do things that, to us, are so obviously a bad idea, but to them . . . who *knows* what will happen?! And as my daughter Turkey will tell you, "Mistakes are how we learn!" How we as caregivers react when they make bad decisions, ask unexpected questions, and push boundaries will impact how safe they feel to come to us for guidance in the future.

So how do we live up to our promise that our love and positive regard for them is unconditional when our children make bad decisions? The model I use for my own children is very much based in what I experienced in my own childhood and young adulthood. Though there are a myriad of examples of this to choose from my earliest (and first) core memory happens to be a great example of both natural consequences and unconditional positive regard.

If you can, imagine a shopping mall in the early '90s. Wait, make that a rural Midwest shopping mall in the early '90s. Way less Day-Glo, way more burgundy and teal. There were only two anchor stores, and the biggest draws were the movie theater and the then thriving craft store. The craft store was really the only reason my mom ever went to the mall—she frequently made clothes for us, as well as quilts and wall hangings that she saw on public access television craft shows. My mom didn't bother with the anchor stores—they were outside the budget and didn't carry clothes that fit her incredibly tall children. No, the mall was really only for craft supplies and the occasional trip to the movie theater.

For my older siblings, however, the mall was a great place to find new music, shoes for various sports, and food. So even though my mother didn't need to venture any farther into the mall than the craft store just inside the main entrance, on one fated trip, after buying my sister some new basketball sneakers, we found ourselves in the heart of the mall. I was roughly four years old, and I had (in my memory) held it together pretty well, given that I had just been forced to sit through my mother's rigorous and extensive shoe selection process. I was granted a walk through a kids' accessory store that for the purposes of this book shall remain nameless (okay, fine, it was Claire's). Everything was fluffy pink, lavender, and baby blue. Earrings shaped like food adorned just about every surface, and there was an entire wall of hair accessories that only the chicest of chic *Tiger Beat* cover models could have pulled off.

I had never been allowed into this store before, or at least I don't remember ever being brought in there until this fateful day. And I may not look it now, but I was *peak* Fancy Kid. I lived for my elbow-length satin gloves and my clip-on earrings. With eyes like dinner plates, I was perusing the irresistible wares with strict instructions to TOUCH. NOTHING. I was a Fancy Kid, but I was also a clumsy one, and it was no stretch of the imagination to envision me tipping over a display or accidentally ripping an entire shelf off the wall.

It's worth mentioning here that one of the ideas that has changed between the way I was parented and the way I parent my children is that "don't" statements have been swapped out for alternatives that include what the child *should* do. The way I phrase it for my own kids, and the rule I would've provided four-year-old me is: "There's lots of breakables in this store, so your hands need to be in your pockets or behind your back." The first few trips with this approach sound like a skipping CD, but once the kids know what's expected of them, they do it with a single reminder.

So, there I was in Claire's, dutifully following the rules, until I saw ... it. The most *beautiful* headband. It was blue, with two little furry puffballs on the end of springs that bobbled around when you put the headband on. I was instantly enamored, and all my impulse control went out the window. In seconds I had the headband in my hands and was preparing to put it on my head. Naturally, at age four, I knew that to put it on my head I needed to make the bottom wide enough to go over my head. I grasped either end of the sparkly blue arch and pulled them apart. With as much force as was required to break a piece of dry spaghetti, the headband snapped in my hands.

I've thought a lot about what makes this a core memory for me—why, when so much of my childhood is foggy in my recollection, does this moment stick out so much? And I think I've figured out why—this moment was the first time I consciously remember considering lying to my mom. She had her back to me—she hadn't seen me touch the headband, and I could've easily put it down in a box that was to my right. But I didn't. I felt safe enough to walk up to my mom and show her that I had broken the headband. And her reaction was exactly what I had expected: I got a brief scolding for choosing to touch the headband after being instructed not to, and I was informed that I would be using some of my "trip money" to pay for it, meaning that I could no longer buy anything from the store.

And I. Completely. Understood.

I did not cry. I did not protest. I was *very* embarrassed as I handed the broken merchandise to the cashier and apologized—I knew I had made a mistake. The cashier reassured me that it was all right, and even told my mom that I didn't have to pay for it. But—and this next part is controversial for some, but I stand by it—my mom said no. "I appreciate the offer, but she needs to pay for at least part of it—she was told not to touch things because she's not always the most careful." She knew that it was a frustrating, embarrassing, and maybe even a little bit sad lesson for me, but I had a history. I wasn't just clumsy—I was her "f*ck around and find out" kid. I thought of myself as the exception—things wouldn't go wrong for me! And often they didn't . . . but I refused to admit that they even could. So this instance of things going sideways needed to be something I remembered. I didn't need to be *ashamed* of it, but I did need to internalize it. That's why she responded the way she did—a reminder of my mistake, and a natural consequence for the choice. That was it. That was the end. I wasn't constantly reminded of it, or spanked, or told I could never go back to Claire's, or screamed at when we got out of earshot of the cashier, or—the worst possible outcome—permanently labeled as a thief or a "naughty kid." I had made a poor choice, but it didn't define me. And I've never forgotten that.

This experience was just the first in a long line of experiences that drove home for me how vital it is that we accurately and fairly respond to our children's mistakes. These reactions will vary by age (and by incident), but they boil down to this: our boundaries and our children's behavior. Think of boundaries like a fence in your brain that marks what you *will* tolerate and what you *won't* tolerate. They are our values that influence how we set our rules and expectations, and how we communicate those rules and expectations. When we discuss boundaries, we often think of phrases like "You can't talk to me like that" or "You can't touch this." However, neither of those statements are boundaries because they are attempting to explicitly control the behavior of someone else. And though we can somewhat control our children's behavior while they're in the earliest parts of their lives, that influence fades quickly and does not have the positive outcomes we hope for.

Instead, boundaries are expressions of what you will accept from another person. "I will not listen to you speak to me like that" or "I will not allow you to touch this." These are expressions of boundaries because they are enforceable by you—you can choose to stop listening regardless of whether the other person is still talking, and you can choose to remove the object that someone is trying to touch. Framing rules and expectations in this way (even if you only do so in your head) helps clarify the real reason why you have set a rule, and may actually help you eliminate unnecessary rules and those that have become a point of unneeded conflict. Additionally, knowing *why* we've set these boundaries and being able to communicate that "why" will help our children decide whether they will choose to respect the boundary or continue to test and resist it.

When a child—regardless of age—tests a boundary, our reaction to their choices can have a long-lasting effect. When your five-year-old tests her newfound ability to write her name . . . on her white bedroom furniture, you might be tempted to yell at her and pair that yelling with a punishment like taking away her bedroom furniture. When we were kids, that would have been presented as a completely acceptable end result—"You can't handle having furniture, so you can't have furniture." While she might not draw on her furniture again, I wager she's also not likely to come to you when she makes a mistake in the future.

If you're trying instead to raise a child who feels comfortable admitting to you when they've messed up, you may want to consider embracing natural consequences. Rather than taking away the furniture, for example, you may require that she spend time scrubbing the marker or pen off the furniture. If this is not the first time she's colored on something not intended for Pint-Size Picasso-ing, you may let her know that the markers and pens have to "live up high" so they can only be retrieved by a caregiver, and must be used under supervision. While she may not be *happy* with either of these outcomes, they are proportionate reactions that, especially when explained, leave a child feeling secure and knowledgeable about the boundaries and rules that shape her world.

In the situation of me at the store, the boundary my mom expressed—"You can't touch anything"—may seem controlling. But upon reflection, the boundary she was setting was "It's my job to raise you to be a functional adult, so I cannot allow you to be reckless with other people's property." Her boundary was there to keep me safe. I have, on more than one occasion, had to haul a child around in a shopping cart because they were overtired and refuse to stay within my eyesight. I've also had to lock down devices and screens because my kids figured out how to get around the parental controls and stayed up way too late. I've *also* had to inform my children that the answer to a question asked by their older sibling is not something they themselves are ready to hear—another way of keeping them safe that we will address in chapter 4. In these situations, I remind my children that my *whole job* as their parent is to love them, keep them safe, and raise them to be functional adults: "I love you too much to let you do this unsafe thing." It's simple, it's to the point, and, again—it's finite. I will very likely have to explain *why* the activity or information they're being denied is unsafe, but this is where that self-reflection of my own boundaries comes into play. Most of the time, I have thought about the situation ahead of time and know exactly why my answer is no.

That's not to say I can stop them from attempting *all* stupid things— sometimes the "f*ck around and find out" approach is the best way to learn. I try to think ahead about the different ways my children will make mistakes and push boundaries as they grow in part because I want to keep my promise to myself to (generally) react with their futures in mind and only prevent them from making mistakes that are truly harmful. As I look back on each of my children's formative years, some mistake patterns seem almost universal. In early childhood, all of my kids proved that small children are egocentric and tethered strongly to "the now." They had no concept of future consequences, and anything they did to hurt me in anger and retaliation was almost invariably rooted in what would hurt them. I've seen more than one art project torn up in a fit of "I'll show *YOU* to tell me to stop coloring!" and I've consoled all three kids as they learned the very hard lesson that ripping up your art really only impacts . . . you.

I've watched my children test the waters of lying—sneaking treats, extra screen time, or a few more minutes of playing instead of doing what they were asked. And I've talked with those same children about trust and how it's both buildable and fragile. That's not to say I call out *every* lie—I don't! There is a certain sense of autonomy and independence that comes from "pulling one over" on your mom, and if my kids can get that sense of satisfaction from a small lie that *doesn't* hurt them or me, I feel like that's a win. If I catch them out in Every. Single. Tiny. infraction or fib, why would they ever trust that I might treat them with grace and kindness when they make a *big* bad choice?

Because those big bad choices can and *will* happen. I remember naively thinking that the bond I had with my eldest child would be much more powerful than all those tropes of the tough teen years . . . and then he turned thirteen. Along with thirteen came pushing curfew. And Incognito Mode. And whispers with friends. And eye rolls. I didn't know how it had happened, but suddenly, when my kid looked at me, it was with a certain level of disdain.

Okay, I say I didn't know how it happened, but I did—like every teenager, his amygdala had outgrown the rest of his brain, as it does in early puberty. The amygdala, one of the parts of his brain responsible for his emotions, was often in the driver's seat. He was living almost entirely out of his emotional brain, and he was reacting with whatever emotion was strongest long before his cognitive brain could catch up and help him regulate. Once I realized that this was happening, things got . . . I'm not going to say a *lot* easier, but they did get easier. When either of us felt ourselves getting heated, we could say "AMYGDALA" and acknowledge that we were being controlled by emotions, not thoughts. Our bond was still strong, and the Foundation of Unconditional Positive Regard that we had built meant that even after slammed doors and yelling fights, we both knew nothing could shake how this mom felt about her child. I also knew that I had a lot of internal work that needed doing—I was reacting (and sometimes overreacting) to him doing things that were completely reasonable for an early teenager to be doing.

When I hit that phase of life with my eldest, I knew I needed to step back and take stock in my values, boundaries, and communication skills. I needed to reflect on why I had the rules I did, what I was expecting from my children, and how I was relaying that information to them. I knew that without understanding why I felt the way I did, I wouldn't be able to continue guiding my kids as effectively as I wanted to. So I thought about it—what *really* mattered to me? What was my guiding mission? And that line of thinking led me to the wish I make in every tunnel, at every wishing well, and on every falling star: that my children grow up to be healthy, happy, and successful adults. And part of that happiness means freeing them (and, by extension, myself) of shame when it comes to making mistakes.

This pre-reflection is very helpful, particularly when it comes to situations that may bring up strong emotions from us; situations that remind us of our own childhoods or traumas. If we have not reflected on our boundaries regarding the birds and the bees, we may find ourselves reacting in a way that undermines our goal of raising children who feel comfortable enough to talk to us about their mistakes and ask us the hard questions.

Take, for example, finding out that your six-year-old has played "doctor" with a same-age friend. The conversation could go a couple different ways:

Scene: At the Playground

"Amanda! What are you and Brian doing up in the castle? You've been up there a long time!"

"We're playing doctor!"

"You're doing WHAT?! Absolutely not! That's gross and naughty and you're NEVER going to play with him again! We're going HOME!"

Amanda has no space to clarify that "playing doctor" means she has wrapped leaves around Brian's "broken arm" and is listening to his heart with her ear on his chest. She doesn't understand in the slightest why her parent has reacted this way, because she lacks the context that when her *parent* was a child, they were spanked after being caught playing a different kind of doctor.

Now imagine that this same parent has reflected on her boundaries and considered what her goals are for raising a child who feels safe asking questions and revealing mistakes:

Scene: Any Home Anywhere

"Amanda? What are you two doing in there? Why are Heather's pants on the ground?!"

"We are playing doctor! I wanted to see her vulva and she wanted to see mine, so we took turns."

"Oh goodness. Well, I know you're curious about other people's bodies, and it's normal to be curious. But remember—your brain is only ready to explore your *own* body right now, not anyone else's. So everyone needs to put their pants back on and we're going to play in the living room until Heather's mom comes back."

In this scenario, Amanda's *developmentally appropriate* curiosity is acknowledged rather than shamed; she is allowed a voice; and she has been redirected into an activity that is more suitable for her brain and her friend's brain. This scenario has also established a boundary that will hopefully help keep her safe in the future—a knowledge that her body is for *her*, especially at this age, and not for *anyone* else. There is also security in knowing that if anyone ever *does* explore her body, she can tell her safe adult with no negative repercussions.

The situations we're most afraid of our children getting themselves into are going to be the greatest tests of our love and respect. We don't *want* to think about our children making the really big mistakes, but let's face it—it could happen. I encourage you to challenge yourself with the difficult task of reflecting on what will test you the most.

Maybe it's finding out your child holds different political views than you do.

Maybe they have changed their spiritual beliefs.

Maybe they love someone you don't approve of.

Maybe they have hurt themselves . . . or are hurting someone else.

Maybe they are actively hurting you.

And then figure out how you can unconditionally love and unconditionally respect your child in those scenarios, while asking yourself what the boundaries are within that love and respect. How can you show up and support your child while also maintaining your own mental and physical well-being? Even though it is likely to be one of the most painful exercises you ever do, I encourage you to think about this, and genuinely know that there is *nothing* your child can do to make you stop loving them. Because that love—and that unconditional positive regard—is tied to trust.

I trust you, my child, to not do something so bad that I ever have to reconsider my love and respect for you, and to come to me when you mess up.

And you can trust me to show up for you, full stop.

CHAPTER 1: IN BRIEF

Unconditional love is expected of parents—many of us choose to be parents, and we love the people we are raising. Expressing this love should happen often and in ways that children can understand at their age level. Unconditional positive regard is different from unconditional love in that it turns an eye to the future by acknowledging the adults our children have the potential to be if they are given autonomy, respect, and boundaries along with that unconditional love.

Key Takeaways

· Young children (under 7) are very literal; children between 8 and 11 can begin to understand more abstract ideas and the perspectives of other people; and children 12 and older can engage with higher-level thinking and logic.

· Because children's cognitive abilities change so much as they grow, ways of expressing love should, too. "I will never stop loving you" may be more understandable for a young child than "I love you to the moon and back" because measurement and distance are concepts they may not grasp yet.

· A fear of making mistakes can stop a child from asking important questions, so as parents we should foster an understanding that mistakes happen and are meant to be learned from.

· Unconditional love and unconditional positive regard happen best when parents and children have healthy boundaries and respect the boundaries of the other people in their lives.

CHAPTER 2

Curiosity

The 1984 *World Book Encyclopedia* was my gateway to the whole wide world. My parents had spent the earliest part of their marriage—from 1970 to about 1980—as broke college students and parents to both their own children and a whole host of foster children. When my mom graduated from her physical therapy graduate program, they decided to splurge and purchase the full *World Book* set and any supplementary books available. It was a beloved collection, and it survived the big move from North Dakota to rural Minnesota where it was at my disposal on the living room bookshelf for my entire childhood. My favorite volume was the one that contained the entry for "human anatomy." Not because it was a super-enthralling read (which I'm sure it was, but I was like . . . six), but because of the diagrams.

See, the edition of the encyclopedia that my parents had purchased included these clear plastic pages that had the various systems of the body printed on them that stacked together to make a whole person. When you peeled back the page that had the external view of the person, you were greeted with the muscular system. Continue turning pages, and you could see the endocrine system, the vascular system, the skeletal system, and the one that fascinated me the most: the reproductive system. I was fascinated by the parts I knew I had—I had heard the word "uterus" when my mom was pregnant with my little brother. But I was even more fascinated with the part I didn't have . . . a penis. There it was, in all its glory—a transparent organ with a clearly defined urethra, testicles, and major blood vessels. As you may have guessed by now, it didn't really look anything like what a human penis looks like in real life. But to a curious kid, it told me just enough—that a penis was Very Different, but human bodies are mostly very much the same.

That curiosity was not necessarily something I was taught—it was innate. Children are naturally curious about the world—they have to be to learn and grow! Babies put a million things in their mouths to learn their texture, taste, and function. Toddlers try climbing, pushing, pulling, tearing, smashing, and a million other verbs to see how they can impact the objects in their world. Preschool and early elementary school children ask a million questions to learn about the mechanisms responsible for everything they didn't realize existed until recently. We are hardwired to want to learn about ourselves, each other, and our world.

While curiosity is a natural drive, it still needs encouragement—especially when it comes to the drive to seek information. Our children are going to ask a million questions, but learning doesn't just happen from asking questions. We also learn through observation and discussion. Even the most boring or mundane activity can be turned into an opportunity to encourage curiosity.

Imagine you are standing in your kitchen, peeling potatoes for dinner while your preschooler plays pretend cook next to you on the floor. You have just a few spuds left when you notice that one has started to sprout and is not suitable to eat. You could just throw away the potato and get on with your task. It would be totally acceptable to do so, especially if you're tired and need to get dinner on the table. But if you have the mental energy, you could use that potato to engage in curiosity with your kid instead:

"Ooooo, bud! Come look at this potato!"

"What am I lookin' at, Mama?"

You could encourage your child to compare (see what is the same) and contrast (see what is different) the sprouted potato with others:

"Well, how does this potato look, and how do the other potatoes I have left to peel look? What is the same? What is different?"

"Hmmm . . . well, they both have kinda brown outsides. They both have little bumpies. They are both bigger than my hands. But that one has a . . . what *is* that, Mama?"

Now you can encourage your child to come up with a hypothesis—an idea that might explain what they are seeing, and a starting point for further experimentation or testing:

"What do *you* think it is, bud?"

"Ummmm, a finger?"

This exercise can go on for as long as you like—you could take it through most of the stages of the scientific method if you wanted to! Asking the child to test their finger hypothesis by seeing if the potato can point to or grab anything. You could have them collect data by identifying all the things a finger can do and seeing how many of them a potato "finger" can do. You could then help them analyze that data and determine that it doesn't seem to be a finger because it lacks the ability to do all the things a finger is able to do.

You can also decide to share the answer with your child—letting them know that while a finger is an interesting hypothesis, what they're seeing is a sprout, and it means both that the potato probably isn't good to eat anymore *and* that if you plant the potato, it could grow into a plant and make new potatoes. Both courses of action are reasonable in part because your end goal of encouraging curiosity has been achieved in either case. I am of the opinion that as a parent, choosing to move through each day with this kind of curiosity has a twofold benefit: First, it encourages your child's natural curiosity and helps them maintain their desire to continue learning about themselves and the world around them. Second, when you are modeling curiosity on a daily basis, it helps them learn what healthy curiosity looks like and how to go about seeking their information in a healthy way.

Modeling is a form of social learning—where people learn by watching other people—first studied in children by Albert Bandura in 1961. What modeling means in the context of this book is that children are watching how parents treat curiosity—how they behave when asked questions, and how they seek to answer their own questions. Children then use those observations as a blueprint for how they should engage with their own curiosity.

There is also a secret, hidden benefit to choosing a life of curiosity—it helps *you* learn new things, too! As we've already discussed, children are going to ask their caregivers as many questions as they feel comfortable with, and many of those questions are going to be about big ideas and how things work. If you choose a life of curiosity—thinking about things that you don't know and looking up the answers for yourself—you can be ready to guide your child through finding answers to their questions. And sometimes, you will be able to supply the answers yourself!

When we practice curiosity ourselves and model the protocol for finding the information we seek, we're also building a sort of mental parachute. We've all been at our "why" breaking point—when our child has asked the question that finally sends us over the edge and we cannot answer any more. We are tired of trying to think of the answers, and we're definitely not in the mood to look things up. If we have modeled for our children how to seek information from reputable sources and to ask interesting questions, we can redirect "why" into other outlets to save our own sanity.

"Why, Mama?"

"Instead of telling you, I want you to try to think of all the reasons that might be why it does that. Then when I'm done going to the bathroom, we can talk about it some more."

Or:

"Why, Mama?"

"We've already talked about why—I want you to think of a different question. Maybe wondering *how* it does that is something you haven't considered doing!"

Having these phrases and protocols at my disposal saves my sanity and helps me maintain the sometimes delicate lines of communication with my children. While I cannot claim that I have never lost my patience and told my children I just need a break from the questions, I try to keep that kind of "answer" to an absolute minimum.

You see, I worry that if we show our children that asking us questions is annoying or burdensome or unappreciated, they may choose to stop asking us questions. And while that might feel good in the short term—I simply do not need to look up the name of that video game character's third cousin's second wife—in the long term, it leaves us with children who do not want to ask us about things they saw on the internet or heard from a kid on the playground. In fact, they may feel like their best source of information *is* the internet or that kid on the playground, and that can have undesirable outcomes.

My "kid on the playground" moment happened when I was about ten years old. I was playing at a park near my childhood home when Sharon, one of the big kids, showed up. It was the heat of August and we were all clambering for either the swings or the slide—anything to get the wind moving on our faces. Sharon, who had just turned thirteen, was recently back from camp and was taking any chance she could to share with all of us kids who had never been to camp (and likely would never be able to afford to go) how cool her experience was.

"Yeah, it was amazing. We slept in cabins and cooked on fires. It was so cool. And there were boyyyyys there."

"BOYS? You went to a camp with girls *and boys?*"

"Uh, duh. I'm way older than you guys."

"Why does it even matter that there were boys there? It's not like you could *kiss* any of them or anything."

"You guys are such babies," Sharon said defensively. "There were boy campers there *and* boy counselors."

The other kids seemed to know this was a Big Deal. I had no clue why this mattered, but I was listening intently to her story at the bottom of the curly slide just the same.

"Yeah, and the boy counselors were soooooo hot. One of them told me I was sexy."

The other girls oohed and ahhed over this information, as if to lament, if only a boy counselor would call *them* sexy, life would be complete!

Sharon continued: "Yeah. And that boy counselor showed me his *sperm*. It was swimming around in his hand."

This caught my attention. Not for the reason that it likely made you stop in your tracks—as an adult reading this book, you're thinking, *Oh my God, if that's true, then that child was abused at summer camp. Did anyone report this? Is she okay?* (From all accounts, this event never took place—she later stated that she made it up because she wanted us to think she was "grown up" after coming home from camp.) No, the reason I was paying even closer attention was that *I knew you couldn't see sperm with the naked eye.* I had read about it in the *World Book Encyclopedia*! I didn't have the guts to call her out—the other kids were taking everything she said as gospel, and I didn't have the social status to go to war with her *and* all those other kids. Instead, I just made a mental note to never believe anything she said ever again.

As an adult, I have wondered about Sharon and her knowledge of the world at thirteen years old: Why did she know the word "sperm" but not how small they were? Why did she know that they "swam" but not that they were not like tadpoles in the palm of someone's hand? And if she wasn't comfortable finding that information for herself, why had no one in her life taught her about how any of that worked? I know now that the answers to all of these questions are likely wrapped up in the stigma around talking about sex and bodies, especially with children.

Curiosity is completely natural, even curiosity about bodies and sex. Our job as caregivers is to ensure that our children's curiosity is guided in the direction that is healthiest for their brain development and that will facilitate their emotional and physical safety. Because curiosity about bodies, both intellectually and physically, isn't inherently sexual—it protects our health, too. Consider how people with breasts are encouraged to do self–breast exams to look for lumps or changes that might be signs of cancer. Think about how we are taught to pay attention to our bowels and take notice if things change as a sign of nutritional demands, developing cancer, or other needs. And think about how we assess our bodies for injuries: "When I press here it's tender, but it wasn't before." Without a healthy knowledge of our bodies when they are functioning at their best, we will be left unaware of changes that could be life-threatening. And how are we going to know our bodies if we are not encouraged to reflect on and explore them?

This exploration starts at a very young age—it is completely normal for a baby to stare at their hands, chew on their feet, or reach into their diaper and grab their penis or vulva. Toddlers and preschoolers continue this exploration and may discover that some sensations feel better than others. As children grow, they will continue to explore their world . . . and their bodies. As I've said before, this exploration is normal and natural, and can be directed into a healthy respect for self. Rather than treating a child's curiosity about their body like something that doesn't exist, acknowledging it and setting boundaries acts as a protective measure, showing the child that you are not going to shame them for being curious *and* that you are there to keep them safe (which we will discuss in chapter 5).

Remaining receptive and setting boundaries for safety is doubly important when it comes to your child's intellectual curiosity. If we have encouraged curiosity in daily life and shown a willingness to answer our children's questions, then we are likely to be at the top of our children's lists of People Who Can Help Me Understand My World. Because, as we know, their world changes *incredibly* fast. They go from "What is this thing?" to "How does this thing work?" and eventually to "How do I make this thing work with someone else?" And if our children are coming to us with their questions, they are less likely to turn to spaces and people that may not have the ability to answer accurately, or, worse, do not have their best interests in mind—their friends, older children, the internet, or unsafe adults. Better that I be the one explaining to my child, accurately and compassionately, what an orgy is, rather than some faceless person on the internet.

A word of caution, though, when it comes to curiosity—the internet is a wild place. Even if your child has very strict and limited access to the internet (like mine), they will still hear things that you never expected—usually from peers whose access is more loosely monitored. Even though I am online *a lot*, some of the songs, sayings, and trends that have made it home with my children have taken me completely by surprise. I've had to google more than one Classic Vine to fully understand what they're saying. Because you may be seeing things that you never thought you would, I think it's worthwhile to familiarize yourself with Incognito Mode on your browser when you are seeking new information online. One rogue keyword typed in a search box, and suddenly you're receiving advertisements left and right for erectile dysfunction . . . and you don't even have a penis. (Yes, this happened to me in the course of writing this book—I'm hoping to spare you the same fate.)

As much as we may not want to admit it, we should also teach our children how to navigate seeking information on the internet. I remember being completely opposed to the idea when my eldest child was in elementary school—if he had questions, he could come to me and I would make sure he got only accurate information! While I hope he will still come to me for the big stuff (as he has in the past), it has been important for us to establish rules and measures regarding information from other places.

Ideally, I would encourage my child to ask themselves these questions before and during any sort of internet search:

- Can I ask my caregiver?
- Can I ask a different safe adult?
- Is there a nonfiction book in the library with this info?
- Do they cite their sources?
- Does it agree with other answers?
- Was it worth it?

You'll note that I said that *ideally* my child would be this reflective while searching. Unfortunately, we do not live in an ideal world—even the list above is not likely to register with many teenagers. So I've come to the conclusion that starting with something that can be repeated and reinforced—a single, simple phrase—is often a better place to start.

Think before you click, and if what you find scares you—stop.

This mantra is repeated over and over as soon as my children gain access to any type of device. The internet is not easy to navigate for accurate, useful, and inclusive information about sex and sexuality, but kids and teenagers don't know that. (And, as mentioned above, the internet can be a minefield even for adults who have years more experience with tech and research.) Much like abstinence-only sex education, asking our children to just . . . not look isn't going to be the most effective way to guide them through seeking their own information. Instead, having an open dialogue about the experience can yield better results. This isn't always an easy feat, but as you'll discover in chapter 12, it is possible.

Beyond teaching our kids how to find information on their own and answer the questions they ask us, we must remember that there are going to be questions they do not even think to ask. Children, especially children who have not reached the early stages of puberty, may be less likely to ask questions about parts they do not have. A child who does not have a penis may be less likely to ask how erections happen, and a child without a uterus may not be curious about periods. This is something to keep in mind as children get older, especially given that as they approach puberty, you will be having discussions about how bodies interact. Without at least a passing knowledge of how most bodies work, it will be that much more confusing when you try to explain how they work *together*. This is yet another reason to normalize conversational curiosity and present interesting facts throughout our day—it helps the child feel comfortable considering information that may not directly apply to them. You can find examples of books that do this really well in the Resources section on page 285.

Providing appropriate biological knowledge about how other people's bodies work can also be a form of protection. When children feel informed—when they feel that they already know how all of the parts work—there is nothing intriguing or forbidden about it. As much as it may terrify us to consider it, there *are* people who can and do weaponize what our children do not know about their own and other people's bodies. Providing age-appropriate information makes it measurably more difficult for an ill-intentioned person to trick your child into a dangerous situation by offering information that feels illicit. No one can look at little Sibley and say, "Oh, you don't know what an erection is? Let me show you . . ."

You have armed them with knowledge of how bodies work and the security to come to you for open, honest answers.

We must also remember that others in society feel it is their duty to influence children to feel like they shouldn't be curious. Having these ideals projected on them may make them worry that their curiosity makes them weird, bad, or wrong, especially if their questions or searches are related to ideas outside what is presented as "normal" in the mainstream understanding. We must remind them that wanting information about how things work does not determine who you are. To put it simply: Curiosity and behaviors in childhood do not necessarily draw a blueprint for a child's future. Playing wedding doesn't mean a child will ever walk down the aisle; pretending to be a farmer doesn't mean they will ever drive a tractor; and playing fashion designer doesn't mean they'll have a debut at fashion week. In the same vein, as NEMOURS KidsHealth states—and in accordance with researchers and pediatric professionals—"Despite myths and misconceptions, there is no evidence that being gay is caused by early childhood experiences, parenting styles, or the way someone is raised." Supporting a child in exploring who they are, how they feel about themselves, and their interactions with the world all while reminding them of your unconditional positive regard for them is vital in keeping open lines of communication and feelings of safety.

Unconditional positive regard and valuing curiosity can manifest in a helpful communication tool for tweens and teens: a Free Pass for questions about bodies. This hypothetical pass is particularly handy when teens start to venture into territory that may have consequences. It works like this:

"I want you to know that as a teenager you have inherited a Free Pass for questions about bodies. What this means is that you can tell me, at any point, that you have a question you need answered, but that you *do not* want to talk about it any further than getting the question answered. Before asking the question, I'll verify with you that the question is not being asked in the context of something harmful or actively dangerous. If you confirm that, then I will answer the question with no follow-up, no matter what the question is. If it becomes clear that I *do* need to be concerned, then I will follow up, but I promise to explain *why* I am concerned and following up."

Providing this card—which, for the record, does not currently exist as a physical card in my house, but I *could* decide to get crafty with it—allows your teenager to know that you value their privacy, respect their autonomy, and trust their judgment. It also helps your teen start to consider information and situations through a lens of safety and adds an introspective step to their knowledge-seeking process. Imagine your fifteen-year-old son comes to you with this scenario:

"Hey, Mom, I wanna use my Free Pass."

"Oh, uh . . . okay. Nothing I need to worry about safety-wise?"

"No. I just want to know."

"Okay. Ask away."

"Is there, like, a practical reason for scissoring?"

TIRE SCREECH SOUND

Okay, your first thought might be, *Where, PRECISELY, did he hear the term scissoring? What is he watching where this is a thing?* Your second thought might be that he really doesn't need to know, because it's not like he'll ever need to do it—he doesn't have a vulva! But if you give yourself a beat, you might realize he is coming to his safest adult to answer a question that is perplexing him *before* he turns to the internet and whatever cursed information he might find there.

"What do you mean by 'practical'?"

"Like . . . is there a reason for it?"

"I mean . . . nothing beyond it feeling good for the people who do it, as far as I'm aware. The same bits are stimulated, no like . . . special spot is activated or anything."

"Oh. Okay . . . thanks."

At this point, you might have to fight the urge to ask why he needs to know—I know my curiosity would be killing me!—but you know that if you violate the terms of the Free Pass, he may never use it again. It might also be tempting to continue the conversation and offer up information that is related and clarifying, but, as we'll cover in the Consent for Knowledge chapter, it's vital to ask if they want the information before going too far into the conversation. Think about where he might have learned the term—is it something he's read online or heard a peer reference, or could it be that he's accessing pornography? Instead of offering up more information, you decide to make a mental note to have a separate talk about relationships, representation, and porn at some point in the near future, but since the question had no super tangible impact on his safety *right now*, you let it go. Consider, however, a slightly different scenario with the same child:

"Mom, I wanna use my Free Pass."

"Reminder of the safety clause!"

"Yeah, I know . . . is it illegal to buy the morning-after pill with a fake ID?"

"Ahhhh. Okay. Well, I'm going to need a little more context, bud, and I can't promise I won't need to follow up, especially if this is about you or someone you know."

"Yeah . . . I kinda figured."

You can compassionately continue the conversation, and if you have done some pre-reflection on how you might handle tough questions like these, you can also give your child an answer while still reminding them of your unconditional positive regard for them. These scenarios are not outside the realm of possibility—every day, teenagers encounter new and sometimes confusing information, scary and life-altering decisions, and the pressure to always know what's up. The very least we, as parents, can do is let them know that we love them enough to help them navigate their ever-changing reality and give them an out when they just can't handle the third degree.

CHAPTER 2: IN BRIEF

Healthy curiosity about ourselves and the world around us is valuable for all humans. Though kids are naturally curious about their world, it's important to help them learn how to seek information that is accurate and appropriate for their developmental age. By guiding our children in their curiosity, we can both answer their questions and help them learn how to safely answer their questions for themselves in the future.

Key Takeaways

- Children are going to be curious about their body, and one of the first ways they are likely to learn about it is by touching it. Setting boundaries about how they can do this safely is important for their health and development.

- It can sometimes feel like our children never stop asking questions. As parents, we can support our children's inquisitiveness and maintain trust by working on our own emotional regulation, so we don't snap when asked a million "whys."

- Acknowledging our children's curiosity and providing accurate, age-appropriate information can help protect our children from people who would seek to exploit their innocence.

- A Free Pass is a tool that shows children they can *always* come to us with questions, even questions they worry are "bad," because we have unconditional positive regard and unconditional love for them.

Consent

My middle daughter, Turkey, has always been the queen of what is known as bodily autonomy. In other words, that girl will not let anyone but herself make any decisions about her body—she is calling 100% of the shots.

One day when Turkey was about three years old, we were doing some shopping at our beloved haunt—Target. We had perused our favorite sections and were making our way through the grocery aisles when we ran into an acquaintance of mine. This nice older woman had never met any of my children and was as charmed by Turkey as most people are.

"Oh my goodness, aren't you a sweet little thing!"

"Nice to meet you."

"And such good manners, too! Oh I just wanna give you a little . . . *boop*"

And she booped my daughter on the nose.

Without missing a beat, Turkey furrowed her eyebrows and poked the woman on *her* nose.

"Oh! My!" said the woman, taken aback that a little girl would poke her in the face.

"Did you like that?" asked Turkey.

"Um . . . I mean . . . ," the woman sputtered.

"Then don't do it to me."

The woman stepped back, a bit bewildered, and walked away without saying much more. Turkey and I just carried on with our shopping. She had handled the situation, so no commentary was needed from me.

I remember telling that story to a friend a few days later and having them raise their eyebrows in alarm. "You let her get away with poking somebody in the face?" she asked me.

"What do you mean 'let her get away with' it? It's her body, and the woman poked her in the face first."

"Well, yeah, but like, it's rude. It was just a boop."

"No. What's rude is that this woman poked her in the face without taking into consideration whether she wanted to be poked in the face—it doesn't matter that it was 'just a boop.' Turkey was just returning the favor."

It's entirely possible that you had the same reaction to reading that story as my acquaintance did. After all, it seems pretty reasonable to say that little kids should not be poking grown-ups in the face, right? Maybe you thought, *She should have just told her to stop,* or *Maybe she should have said "Next time, ask first," and that would have been enough.* And I counter with this: At three years old, how many people do you suppose listen to Turkey? (Other than her immediate family, of course, who almost always listened to three-year-old Turkey.) The unfortunate answer is that because of her age, not a ton of people listened. Using her words might have worked to stop the interaction—it's possible. But poking this woman in the face absolutely worked. Turkey set a boundary for her body—*I will not let you poke my face*—and provided a very concrete demonstration of what would happen if the boundary was violated—she'll poke you back.

We established in chapter 1 that kids don't understand abstract thought until they're getting close to their teen years. That's the whole reason why we use very concrete statements like "There's nothing you can do to make me stop loving you." Starting as soon as they're able to understand the spoken word, we want to keep things clear, concise, and easily understood. Unfortunately, consent is one of those concepts that can easily get abstract if we let it, because a lot of factors influence what counts as consent. That's why for small children, we use both the word "consent" and a catchphrase similar to the one we use for love. For my family, our consent and bodily autonomy phrase is "It's my body and I get to pick." The phrase still fits firmly within consent because making choices about what you will allow to be done with and to your body is the definition of consent. However, by clearly stating "It's my body and I get to pick" rather than using just the word "consent," we consistently reinforce and help the child internalize the fact that consent means they get to say yes *and* no.

Now, before we go much further, I want to make something very clear: "It's your body and you get to pick" only applies in situations that are not health and safety related. It's your body, but you do not get to pick if you wear a seat belt. It's your body, but you do not get to pick if you are clean. It's your body, but you do not get to pick whether you will be getting your broken arm set with a cast. Sometimes there are situations where your safe adult has to step in and make sure that you are being cared for in the way that helps you grow and stay healthy.

It's helpful to consider what your health and safety nonnegotiables are for your child before you ever get to the point where they might argue with you about them. For me, my nonnegotiables are almost entirely safety related, and include holding hands in parking lots, being within eyesight while out in public, remaining buckled in when in a car, bathing routinely, getting annual blood draws (if required), and brushing hair. Now, some might argue that brushing hair is not a health or safety standard, but I disagree. My children's hair texture requires regular brushing if they are going to wear it long because it can become matted; collect dirt, mold, and mildew; and just generally negatively impact their health and well-being. That doesn't mean I hold them down and brush their hair. It simply means that they have a choice: They can either have their hair brushed (by me or by themselves), or they can choose to have shorter hair. One or the other.

See, even within safety requirements there can be autonomy via choice. You can choose whose hand you'll hold in the parking lot. You can choose to walk near me, in my eyesight, or ride in the cart. You can choose to buckle yourself in or let me buckle you. You can choose a bath or a shower. You can choose what color bandage you'll get after your blood draw. Empowerment in exercising bodily autonomy can happen within the boundaries of health and safety.

In situations that are not health or safety related, my children have autonomy over their bodies. Hugs, kisses, tickles, wrestling, pats on the backs, or physical ways of getting their attention (like being poked)—my children get to choose what kinds of and how much touch they will accept. I have one child who loves getting tickled everywhere except the bottoms of their feet.

They have made it abundantly clear that they would love to get tickled all the time, so long as you don't touch the bottoms of their feet. I have another child who loves to be tickled, but only with what they call tiny tickles. No big belly scratches that make them double over—they want little bitty tickles in very short bursts. Again, please tickle them as much as they want, but only with tiny tickles. They get to decide what kind of and how much touch they receive at any time.

As humans, we communicate verbally and nonverbally, and within that communication there are almost countless variations of inflection, word choice, body language, proximity, and other factors that can change the meaning of what is being conveyed. We've all heard that no means no, and I think all of us would agree with that. But . . . I'm a Midwesterner. Here "No, yeah" means something different than "Yeah, no." Someone in a movie might say, "No! I can't believe they did that." A sarcastic "no" might actually mean "yes." Upon reflection, we recognize there are countless ways a word as seemingly simple as "no" can be used. That's why we've come up with boundary phrases specifically around physical touch in our home. It's a given that we pause play and check in when someone says "no" or "stop," but the most powerful boundary phrase is "I don't want to play that game." It is an instantaneous hard stop to any activity. The phrase also prompts anyone involved to touch base and find out what's going on: "Okay! Is there a reason you don't want to play this game anymore? Are you feeling done? Are we doing it wrong? Is there something you want to change?" It encourages communication about the situation and models boundary setting—*I as a person am not willing to be touched any more.*

As children get older and their vocabularies increase and they begin to engage with logic and more abstract thinking, we can help them broaden their understanding of and deepen their appreciation for consent. The current gold standard for conceptualizing consent is the FRIES acronym, devised by Planned Parenthood:

F is for freely given.
R is for reversible.
I is for informed.
E is for enthusiastic.
S is for specific.

This acronym helps our children begin to understand the nuances of "I don't wanna play this game." That their "yes" to play any given game is based on a few specific factors.

> **Freely given** means that there cannot be any sort of threat, coercion, convincing, or other circumstance that has made someone say yes when they normally would not. As kids get older, they will learn that individual factors will influence whether consent can be freely given— factors like whether there is power imbalance, whether either party is under the influence of drugs or alcohol, or whether one of the people is cognitively vulnerable.

> **Reversible** means that just because you've said yes before, or even that you said yes 30 seconds ago, does not mean

your yes has to be maintained. You can change your mind at any point, and once you have, the interaction needs to stop.

Informed refers to the information provided about what the person is being asked to consent to. When children are young, it means the difference between big tickles and tiny tickles. But as kids get older and begin to engage with other people, the *I* means asking things like "Are we going to first base or second base?" or "What's your STD or STI status?" and other such questions. Without having all the information about what an interaction might entail, you cannot truly give consent.

Enthusiastic is related to the state of mind of the individual who is providing consent. I don't want you to give me a hug because you feel obligated to—I only want a hug if you want to give me one. Children who are shown that their enthusiasm matters internalize that any interactions between bodies should make both people feel good.

Specific means the consent a person provides only extends as far as it has been defined in the "informed" part of consent. You've agreed to give me a hug. That doesn't mean I can give you a kiss without asking. In their futures, it means they know that just because they've agreed to make out with their partner doesn't mean they have agreed to be naked while they do it.

Respect for consent and bodily autonomy is part of the bedrock of being a safe adult. If you're reading this book, I will be honest with you: I'm assuming that you are a safe adult for children. You respect their autonomy, you listen to their voices, you trust them when they tell you things, and you would never ask them to keep secrets, particularly ones that would make them unsafe. I list all those criteria because those are the criteria of a safe adult. I'm using the term "safe adult" instead of "trusted adult" because unfortunately, most children who experience abuse by adults are abused by someone they know and trust.

I advocate that each child should have least three safe adults they can turn to with questions. I say three simply because of the rule of three, or *omne trium perfectum*—people (kids included) tend to remember lists that contain three items. It's important, too, that children have multiple safe adults they can go to if they need help. These are both true and sometimes difficult to achieve. The world can be a scary place—there are people out there who do not have any scruples about hurting a child. When our children are young, we choose their safe adults for them. We do so by making sure we share very similar boundaries and values, we know that the individual would never lie to us about the situations our children are in, and we've observed how they handle our children's autonomy. We also must acknowledge that children have a say in who their safe adults are—if our kids ever raise a red flag about an individual who has previously been deemed safe, our first priority is to listen. Reversibility in consent extends to picking safe adults, too.

Just like it is important for us to be able to identify a reliable and accurate source of information online and to teach our children that skill, it's important for us to be able to identify who safe adults are and teach our children how to do the same. As their communities grow wider with age, so too will their access to other safe adults. Our children may find a coach, a teacher, a spiritual leader, or the older sibling of a friend who they feel is a trustworthy addition to their cadre of safe grown-ups, and it is their right to do so. If we want to make sure they are adding truly safe people to their social support network, then we have to explicitly spell out to our children what qualities make a safe adult:

> **They make you feel safe.** The most essential part of a "safe" adult is that they make you feel safe. You know that they will not hurt you or ask you to do things that hurt you. They will not put you in situations where you can be harmed, and you know you can trust them.
>
> **They follow the family safety rules.** Safety rules are going to vary by family based on location, size, culture, and demographics. The family safety rules should be explicitly explained, and the nonnegotiable rules should be so clear that any member of the family can recite them

on command. (An example might be "No one picks you up except Mom. If someone else shows up, they have to know the family password.") These safety rules should always include some variation of "No one may touch you in your swimsuit parts, and if anyone does or asks to, you need to tell Mom."

They don't ask you to keep secrets. Safe adults don't ask you to keep secrets, and never threaten you as a way to force you to keep a secret.

They listen to you. Safe adults listen to what you have to say, and they listen to you without judging you or making you feel bad for sharing with them.

Now, you likely noticed above that I talked about "swimsuit parts." You'll find as you go through this book that I almost exclusively utilize biological terminology, and I do not shy away from using the correct anatomical terms for body parts. That holds true when I'm speaking to children, too. That being said, I also use the term "swimsuit parts" when talking to children. People who choose to harm children are savvy, and it is not outside the realm of possibility that someone would use different terminology or slang words to trick a child into complying with predatory demands: "Oh, I know I can't look at your vulva, but your pussy is okay . . ." Absolutely not. By stating the health and safety boundary that "No one should look at or touch your swimsuit parts," a parent provides a concrete, visual representation informing the child that anything covered by a swimsuit is off-limits. It doesn't matter what slang term might be used or any other way it's framed. "My mom says no one should touch me on my swimsuit parts, and that's a swimsuit part."

You also noticed part of picking a safe adult is establishing a strict rule around secrets. Now, I have my fair share of secrets—there are things that even my closest friends do not know about me. As an adult, I am allowed to have secrets. Teenagers are allowed to have secrets from their parents and from their friends. Young children, however—particularly those still in the preoperational stage of development, or under age seven—should never be asked to keep secrets, because dangerous people might frame abuse as a "secret."

Let's say you buy your spouse a really expensive blouse for Christmas and your child sees it. "Hey, that's a secret. Don't tell Mommy" may seem like a natural thing to say. Unfortunately, there is hidden subtext in that request. It implies "Your mommy *shouldn't* know about this, and if you tell her, I'll be upset." A secret implies "If you tell, there might be a bad consequence, and I don't want you to tell anyone."

Instead, consider what the subtext might be with this phrasing: "Hey, that shirt is a surprise, and we get to give it to Mommy at Christmas." Do you see the difference there? The underlying message is "Hey, your mommy *will* know about this, and it's going to be a nice thing for her." There is no threat of consequence, because in all honesty, there shouldn't be one. If the child accidentally spills the beans and ruins the surprise, it's disappointing, but generally not life-ruining. If what a child is being asked to keep hidden *would* ruin someone's life, it is worth reflecting on *why* the child needs to know this information.

You can take the idea of "surprises, not secrets" one step further by sharing surprise planning with them . . . and planning surprises for them. I'm personally a big believer in throwing my children at least one surprise party so they know what it feels like to have a good surprise. I want them to know that surprises are positive, joyous things that are designed to make people feel good—so that if anyone asks them to keep a "secret" that they feel might be unsafe, their alarm bells will go off.

Though we strive to choose the safest people to be near our children, and to teach our children how to identify who is and isn't safe, we cannot guarantee that we will have 100% success, as much as it pains me to say. As you saw earlier in the chapter, our children can get their boundaries tested directly in front of our faces. And we won't always be there with our children—people who aim to hurt children are very good at putting themselves in situations where they have the chance to do so. As a result, one of the most important parts of protecting our children's safety is, again, unconditional positive regard: reminding your child that not only is there nothing they can do that will make you stop loving them, but also that you *believe what they tell you, the first time they tell you.* Even if you feel you have to investigate, even if your child has a history of spinning yarns or spouting tall tales, even if you think there's no *way* what they're saying is right—your first reaction is "Thank you for telling me." Because keeping them talking, keeping them telling you, is parenting with an eye to their future.

CHAPTER 3: IN BRIEF

Consent is a concept that can be modeled and taught beginning when children are infants and toddlers. They can be shown that they have a say in how their body is treated, and they can learn the evolving boundaries of their own autonomy at the same time. Conversations about consent, both as it applies to children and to their interactions with others, must be ongoing, because of how children's cognitive abilities change as they grow.

Key Takeaways

- Consent often starts as questions about what a child will or won't engage with physically. Asking permission for hugs, tickles, cuddles, and other forms of physical engagement allows a child to practice giving and revoking consent.

- Consent is important, but it does not supersede a child's health and safety. Reflecting on what you consider health and safety non-negotiables will be helpful when discussing and practicing consent with your child.

- It's helpful to establish boundary phrases like "I don't want to play that game" or "I will not let you tickle my feet" with your child so that setting and maintaining boundaries can become comfortable.

- The safe adults in your child's life must understand and respect consent, and choosing safe adults includes having conversations about values, boundaries, and consent.

CHAPTER 4

Consent for Knowledge

My mom did an excellent job of showing me how loved I was growing up. I didn't fear making mistakes, and when I asked questions, I was confident that the answers she gave me were scientifically accurate. After all, I had unrestricted access to a whole suite encyclopedia (which, as you learned earlier, I took *full* advantage of) and The Learning Channel was frequently the channel of choice in our house—my favorite was watching total knee replacements. Heck, my mom even took advantage of one of her own injuries to teach us about the anatomy of the inner arm.

My parents had purchased their first-ever home when we moved to the small town where I grew up. It was a story-and-a-half house with bedrooms over the garage and a couple sets of stairs up to the front door. After living in the house for almost a decade, my mom declared that the wrought-iron front railing needed to be painted to deal with the rust after harsh Minnesota winters. She dutifully took the railing down and spread it out in the garage to be sanded and painted. Later that week, after putting on the first coat of paint, she needed to run an errand, so she hustled inside and grabbed her purse.

As she walked out the front door and headed down the stairs, she tried leaning on the . . . nonexistent railing. Naturally, because there was nothing there to support her, she went "ass over teakettle" (her words) and fell to the landing. She gathered her wits, noticed *some* blood, and came inside to holler for my dad. After grabbing a flour sack towel from the kitchen to stanch the bleeding, she headed back out the front door to go to the car. As she walked past the living room, she was met with the stunned faces of my older sister, myself, and my little brother.

"Oh, hi, kids. I fell down."

"Clearly," my sister replied somewhat sarcastically.

"Yes, well, I'm headed to the hospital."

"WHY?!" I asked, a rather silly question, given that she was leaving drips of blood on the tile.

In an attempt to reassure me, my mom launched into an explanation . . . and an anatomy lesson.

"Well, you see, when I fell, the corner of the step cut my arm. See the blood? Well, under the blood you can see the muscles that make up my wrist flexor group, and some fat, and if you look closely . . . here, you can see the bone! So I'm going to head to the doctor so they can sew my arm back up and put a bandage on it. You stay here with your sister."

The child was too stunned to speak.

My mom headed out the door and got her stitches, and I sat on the couch, processing. I had asked a question and gotten an answer . . . though not necessarily the one I was expecting. I don't fault my mom for giving me what some could argue was a little too much information—she was in a bit of a state, so her judgment maybe wasn't perfect—and the result has made for great family lore.

This was an instance where *normally* my mother would have asked for consent to give me this knowledge. At any other time, when we asked questions that might be answered with scary or overwhelming or really just a lot of information, my parents would verify that we actually wanted to know. This verification came in several forms, but the simplest and most straightforward was directly asking us "Are you sure you want to know?" As a parent, I have maintained this method, but with a slight change: I include the reason why I'm asking.

"Mom, how do the cells get *in* a uterus to make a baby?"

"That question has a couple different answers, might make you think of more questions, and will probably make you feel some pretty big and interesting feelings. Are you sure you want to know right now? Or would you like to wait?"

My kids have taken every possible route when asked this question, from asking to wait until later all the way to insisting on knowing and asking several follow-up questions. But in every scenario, they have felt in control and able to steer how much they were learning, all because they have given consent for knowledge. They have felt empowered to direct the conversation and to tell me when they wanted more information and when they were ready to disengage. The idea that your child can basically ask you to shut up might feel off-putting, but think about how many times you have looked away from a news story or opted not to open a comment thread online. When we are a primary source of information for our children, I believe they need to have the option to "close window."

See, when we talk about consent, it is almost always framed in the physical sense. Chapter 3 stressed how important it is to teach our children that they have the ability to give and withdraw consent over their own bodies, and that they must obtain consent when interacting with other people's bodies. But very infrequently do we consider teaching children (or anyone, really) about consent in the mental, emotional, or spiritual sense.

At the beginning of this book, I recounted how my dad sat me down to have The Talk and revealed that I remember very little of it. I am fairly certain that part of the reason my brain kicked up the '90s pop to drown out my dad was that I had not consented to hear the information he was presenting. Not because it was new information, but because I was not in a mental or emotional place to want to hear it from my *dad*. I had already reached the point in our relationship where we could *joke* about bodies and sex—he got me good when we were watching *Ghost* and during the pottery scene simply said, "You know what that is supposed to stand for, right?"—but having a frank and open conversation about things my body might feel and how I might someday date? Absolutely not. I was not in a place to have that conversation . . . but he didn't ask. And I think he was so intent on giving the lecture correctly that he couldn't see that I wasn't listening.

The most important thing to remember as you embark on having these conversations is just that—they are *conversations*, not lectures. These are opportunities to sit down and share information, yes, but also to listen to what your child has to say about what they may or may not know. To get a read on their feelings toward relationships, sex, and themselves. On balance, you should be listening at least as much as you are talking, if not more. Because if you're not listening . . . then they likely aren't, either.

That is not to say that we should let the conversation die if they are not talking—this information is too vital for us to simply skip it. We need to become facilitators of conversation, learn to ask questions and ease discomfort so our children feel empowered to discuss with us or to seek information in other safe places. One of the most powerful questions you can ask your child is "What do you want to know?" Even though it is six simple words, it can be used for several different purposes:

"Mom, what is an orgy?" asks Rick, age fourteen.

"What do you want to know?"

"Well, what is it?"

"Okay. It's when a group of more than three people have sex."

"Oh. Uh. Okay."

In this scenario, the question was answered in the simplest and most straightforward way because the child confirmed that they wanted an operational definition—what is it? And given their age and previous knowledge, it's important for them to have the information and follow the "asked and answered" mantra. But there are other ways a similar situation could go, especially with different ages:

"Dad, can you tell me about an orgy?" asks Monica, age eleven.

"What do you want to know?"

"Um, well, what is it?"

"The answer might make you have a lot of complicated feelings. Are you sure you want to know?"

"Oh . . . uh . . . well . . . maybe?"

"Hmmm. Sounds like you're not sure. What do you *want* to know?"

"I guess I just want to know if it's something that teenagers actually do."

"I can tell you that *most* teenagers are not doing it, and that if a teenager *is* doing it, I have some concerns. Would you like to use your Free Pass?"

"No, I'm good. I just figured out that Jared is probably full of crap."

"I'm not going to ask, but if it's Jared P. talking about orgies, you're right—he's probably full of crap. When you feel like you're ready for more info, I'll tell you, and you'll know I'm right."

In this scenario, the child made it clear that they didn't really want all the details, but they did need to know enough to ease their minds and make sure they didn't feel out of step with their peers. By changing the tone of the question and making it clear that the child was in the driver's seat on the information bus, the conversation went where it needed to go.

Intellectual consent, or consent for knowledge, follows the same rules as physical consent, so it can be revoked at any time. It is very empowering for a child to know that they can not only stop listening, but tell you to please stop talking when they are feeling done with a conversation.

At a truck stop late one evening, I was reminded of the joys of having a new reader in my household. We had gone in to use the restroom and my daughter was standing by the sink waiting for everyone to finish drying their hands so we could hit the road. As she stood there, she caught sight of a sign advertising help for victims of human trafficking.

"Mom . . . what is sex-you-all assault and human . . . whatever that said?"

"Sexual assault and human trafficking?"

"Yeah, that's it."

"Oh boy. Where did you see those words?"

"On the sign in the bathroom."

"Okay, well, are you sure you want to know? It might make you have a lot of questions, and these answers might be a bit scary."

"I do want to know."

At that point, I explained the concept of rape to my nine-year-old child. I explained that sometimes, people will hurt other people with sex. That when a person violates another person's consent and does things to their body without permission, that's called sexual assault. That this hurts the person, and that people who have been sexually assaulted or raped deserve to have support and help in recovering from that hurt. And then I checked in.

"I know that's a lot to learn about—if you want to take a pause in talking about it for now, we absolutely can."

She opted to take a pause—she needed time to process that contrary to her life experience so far, not everyone asked for consent or respected other people's boundaries. Her face was fixed up in concern and deep thought, so I made sure to reassure her with a mantra we've used for her whole life.

"Hey, kiddo—you remember that my whole job is to keep you safe, right?"

"Yes."

"What happens if anyone tries to push your boundaries or not wait for your consent?"

"I . . . say no? Don't let them?"

"You can say no, that's true. But what else? You tell . . ."

"Mom."

"And what will Mom do?"

"Protect me."

She had asked me a question, provided her consent to receive the information, and then withdrawn consent when she realized she wanted more time before engaging with the information further. For *my* child in *this* moment with *this* subject, I felt comfortable allowing her to be the judge of what she was ready for. But being willing to provide the information simply because I was asked is not always what happens—just as it's our job to protect the physical safety of our children, it's our job to protect their intellectual and emotional safety, too.

If my five-year-old had been awake when my older child asked the question about sexual assault and human trafficking, my answer would have been different. My answer would have been: "I know you want to know what those concepts are, but your little sister is not old enough to understand them yet. So to keep her brain safe, we are going to wait to talk about them until we have some privacy." These limits—a willingness to say "Your brain isn't ready for this, but I'll write it down and we'll talk about the things you need to know *before* I explain what you're asking about"—extend to topics we don't feel our children have the foundation to understand yet.

As a caregiver, you know your children very well. You know what brings them joy, you know what makes them sad, you know how they handle being scared, and what makes them laugh. You also know if they can hold information separately in their minds, or if they tend to catastrophize. I have answered questions differently depending on how the child asking handles information. I have one child who is basically the physical manifestation of anxiety—they are quick to jump to what *could* go wrong, and any negative happenings in the world can easily be thought of as happening to *them*. In contrast, another child is much better at understanding that bad things happen, *and* that they are not terribly likely to happen to *them*. These differences in our children are why it's important to remember that all the guidelines set out in this book are exactly that—guidelines.

There's no one "right" age for giving children information. And there's no perfect formula for knowing if a child is ready to hear things. We might make mistakes—we might think a child isn't ready, only to discover they already know. Or we might think that because our child asked, they are ready to hear it . . . when in reality, they are trying to process something they were inadvertently exposed to. Just like the Bob Ross analogy at the beginning of this book, we can take errors in judgment and turn them into "happy accidents"—take our inevitable missteps in our sharing of knowledge and recover from them. Simply making a mistake in how we have or have not shared information doesn't make the overall work we've invested invalid or ruin our child's future. What is important is that we communicate honestly with our kids regarding what they know and want to know, think carefully about our boundaries regarding sharing information, and feel comfortable and prepared to enforce those boundaries when our kids test them.

Because boyyyyyy, will they test them.

By asking you questions you never saw coming.

Questions like "Did you and Uncle Jeff have sex?" when you and your brother-in-law emerge from a room with a closed door.

Or "Did Mom have lubrication when you made me?"

Or "If you go on a date with that person, will you have sex with them?" ·

Kids. Are. Curious. They are trying to figure out the world, and for a big chunk of their early life, you are really their only reference point. They are going to try to get as much information out of you as they can . . . and you don't have to provide it.

> "Hey, that's a private question and I'm not going to tell you about if I have sex."

> "It's generally considered rude to ask people about how they have sex or what their sex was like."

Just like your children have the right to consent to *receiving* knowledge, you have to consent to *providing* it. You can decline to provide answers for any number of reasons: it is private information about you; it's information that they do not have the required basic information to understand; the answer will be harmful or scary for them to hear.

If you do not think a child is prepared to hear the answer to their question, it might be tempting to probe why they know enough to ask it. Terrifying thoughts might be racing through your brain—who hurt your baby so they know that? It *is* valuable to find out where they got information you didn't provide them—you need to know if there is something harmful happening or if someone is being careless with what they access in front of your child—but it is also valuable to maintain comfort when discussing these sensitive topics.

Instead of grilling your child for information or letting on that you are scared that they know these words, approach fact-finding with humor.

"Psh, *that's* a heck of a word! Where did you hear *that!?*" said with a laugh will likely elicit a much different response than a panicked "Tell me why you know that word!" Once you have the answer to the question, knowing how to proceed becomes much clearer.

> "Oh, you read that word in one of my romance novels? Well, I know you are able to read them now, but those books have content that your brain is not quite ready for. If you want to read about people falling in love and all of that, we can get you some books that are written for kids your age. They probably have a bunch of *kissing* in them and everything!"

> "Ahhh, your brother was playing video games and you heard another player in the lobby call someone that? I'm going to remind your brother that he needs to have his volume turned down and that he needs to be muting people who talk like that. That word is a grown-up word, and it's also very rude to call other people that word."

> "Thank you for telling me. Those kinds of movies aren't made for kids your age, and your grandma shouldn't be watching them while she's watching you. I'm very proud of you for telling me and helping me keep your brain safe."

In none of those situations did a child hear information they weren't prepared to hear. Instead, their caregiver set a boundary (*I will not share that information with you*), informed the child *why* that information wasn't being shared (*the information is not suitable for you to have yet*), and reassured the child that *they* were not the reason the information was being denied. Remind the kid that the most important thing is their safety, and that sharing the information with them at that time is not a good way to keep them safe, while also keeping the door open for future conversations. It's not that the child *shouldn't* know the information, it's that they shouldn't know it *yet*.

Our willingness to set the boundary of what we will and won't answer for our children is also vital modeling for our children, because as we know—kids talk. Kids want to know the answers to all the questions. "Where did that come from?" "How did you get that?" "When did that happen?" And on and on. If we are the kind of parents who are going to share our knowledge, we must also help our kids know when they should and shouldn't share *their* knowledge.

Kids trying to figure out their world will seek information from any source they can. For children who have their questions answered honestly, having a boundary phrase is helpful for when their peers start asking them questions. In my family, the phrase is "Ask your safe adult." I remind my children frequently that just because they have this information doesn't mean that somebody else's parents want them to have the same information. That's not our choice to make. "If your friends ask you questions, even if you know the answer, the answer has to be 'you need to ask your safe adult.'"

This guideline does become a little bit relaxed as kids get older—when children begin dabbling in romantic relationships, they *must* share information with their partners to protect everyone's safety—but children who are in middle childhood or the preoperational stage of development should deflect questioning. Children who are just learning the very basic mechanics of where babies come from are not educated enough to accurately answer the questions of their peers, and as such, the answer is always "Ask your safe adult."

Consent for knowledge is also heavily impacted by how you present the information and what kind of kid you have. When my mom fell down the stairs and gave me an impromptu anatomy lesson, it was because she has a penchant for gravitas. She takes biology very seriously and believes that all human body topics should be treated with the utmost respect. And I appreciate that about her a lot, but sometimes you just need to laugh about the absurd stuff that bodies do. Sometimes the only way to feel normal about something that is "normal-adjacent" is to laugh about it. That is to say, how we *present* information can make a big difference in how our kids receive it.

One of my very favorite people had a sticky penis when he was younger. Before you get weirded out, what I mean is that his penis had adhesions. He was uncircumcised, so when he would try to retract his foreskin, it would get stuck. For the most part, this didn't cause him much issue . . . until he hit puberty. When he needed to be able to retract his foreskin for things like cleaning, enjoyment, and self-exploration, he was having a lot of pain. And when he was twelve, his doctors determined that for the health of his penis, he needed to be circumcised.

Naturally, this was a big freaking deal. And mixed in with the nerves and the discussion about healing time, there was some embarrassment. Thankfully, this person had probably the coolest older sister in the history of older sisters, who happens to be a very dear friend of mine. She knew that her little brother needed humor to cope with this ordeal, rather than discussing it with grave seriousness. Though he was a very serious kid in a lot of ways, he didn't need that kind of tone when approaching this particular experience.

He needed it normalized, especially because there were going to be questions from his peers in the locker room after soccer. She knew she had to take some of the seriousness out of the experience and add a little bit of humor and casualness. And she did that . . . with Frankenweenie.

She made jokes about his post-surgery "Frankenweenie." She talked about Frankenweenie. She asked how Frankenweenie was doing. Sometimes she would refer to how people might scream if Frankenweenie were to come alive like Frankenstein's monster. This was the perfect level of juvenile humor for a twelve-year-old recovering from a circumcision. And it was the exact armor he needed when, inevitably, his peers made some comment about him being a bit of a freak for having to have "dick surgery." He'd already made all the Frankenweenie jokes; he didn't need to worry about what his weird peers would say.

One of the final aspects of consent for knowledge is acknowledging that we aren't always the ones our kids want their answers from. Sometimes, our kids just don't wanna freaking talk to us. Though our family strives to have an environment of open, safe communication, there are some things my kids just don't want me to know about them, and that's okay. There are sex topics I just don't want to talk about with my mom. So how could I possibly feel that my teenager should have to hear everything from *only* me? Surrounding our children with a community of safe adults and resources that are accurate and reliable is a great way to make sure they are getting the information we want them to have, even if they don't want to ask us. Giving our children an out—another adult or adults, books, keywords, safe search advice, etc.—lets them know that we trust them, and we respect them, and we know they are competent to give their consent for knowledge.

CHAPTER 4: IN BRIEF

Though consent is most often discussed in a physical sense, consent for knowledge is also a valuable concept. Learning new information can elicit strong emotions, particularly when the information is surprising or unexpected. In children, these strong emotions may result in a child no longer wanting to seek information or feeling like they have done something wrong by asking a question. Consent requires that both parties be fully informed, so consent for knowledge acknowledges the potential outcomes of sharing information in order to provide informed consent.

Key Takeaways

- "If a child is old enough to ask, they're old enough for an answer" does not account for the source of the question or the emotional preparedness of the child.

- When an elementary school–age child asks a question that may have a surprising or scary answer, informing them of the potential outcome provides them the opportunity to opt out of hearing that answer.

- A child being able to disengage from an upsetting conversation is similar to an adult choosing to stop watching a scary movie or taking a break from reading upsetting news. It does not mean the child will avoid the topic forever—it means the child is protecting their mental well-being in that moment.

PART 2

MECHANICS (BIRTH TO AGE 10)

The idea of talking to your child about body parts that you yourself do not have can feel intimidating. You wonder, *How can I possibly be accurate in my explanation and empathy when I don't understand at all what it's like to have one of those?* One of the questions I'm asked most is "How do I approach body talk with my child when their anatomical makeup doesn't match mine?" I have heard so many stories from people who have asked someone else—a friend, a family member, or, most often, the other parent—to explain the facts to their child, only to find out later that just having the same bits didn't make the experience much easier, and the child is just as mystified as they were before.

It's clear to me that parents are worried they are going to make mistakes—that they are either going to overexplain or underexplain something and end up doing damage to their child. In an attempt to avoid the damage, they do one of two things—they either put the topic off for later, or they pass the child and their questions along to someone else.

Putting the topic off isn't inherently bad—if you need time to look up information and gather your wits so you can accurately answer your child's question, then by all means, take the time you need! But if the parent is putting off the topic in the hope that their child will forget or that they will find the information elsewhere (the alternative source I hear most often is "in-school sex ed"), then there is increased risk that the child will feel they can no longer seek information from their caregivers, leaving them vulnerable to getting inaccurate information, or, worse, harmful information from someone who seeks to hurt them. This is not outside the realm of possibility, especially considering that comprehensive, accurate sex education and healthy relationships education is not the norm in the US, and is indeed only required in SEVEN states, while twenty-two states require that abstinence be stressed.

It is also not inherently bad to ask for help in explaining topics that you have not and will never experience. As I mentioned, I will always and forever advocate for children to have at least three safe adults who they can go to for questions. It's hard to stomach sometimes, but I know I will not be my children's first choice for some questions—they don't necessarily want me to know all of their business, and privacy is their right. So if there are other adults whom you trust to tap in to provide information for the safety of your child, then you should include them in your child's emotional and intellectual safety net. If "Hey, Mom, why do I have a long penis?" is something you think your husband would explain better, then you can feel free to say, "Well, sweetheart, it's called an erection, and your dad can help you understand what to do when it feels like that." And if you as a dad discover that your daughter has had a leak of menstrual blood on her sheets overnight, it's okay to help her change the sheets and recommend that she discuss with her mother how to prevent it from happening again.

But sometimes Dad isn't available, and sometimes Mom isn't around. Sometimes we are the only and best option for our children to seek information, and as our children's first and best defense against harm, we need to arm ourselves with information and confidence when it comes time to explain these sensitive topics. Information and confidence are what the following chapters are here to help you build. Discussing the mechanics of the body—from an individual level—is where body talk starts. Helping you and your child understand how it all works as their bodies grow and change, from exploring and understanding what each part of the body does all the way to discussing how bodies can work together to make new life. It's this simple: We should be able to explain all their parts as comfortably and accurately as we would explain their elbows.

CHAPTER 5

Self-Stimulation and Exploration

"Now that you have your period, you'll want to make sure that you're washing yourself well. Don't use soap because it's not good for your vagina, but you can take the showerhead down and use the warm water to rinse everything off."

I keep saying I don't remember much from my childhood, but I remember this.

Great, I thought, *more crap to do in the shower. My hair is already so hard to wash—this is just another annoying thing to do.*

I have never asked my mother if she knew what she was doing, in part because I don't feel like I need to—I believe she absolutely knew what she had done for me. You see, when I first took down the showerhead with the intention of washing myself more thoroughly, I had no idea what I was in for.

It. Felt. Great.

This isn't *that* kind of book, so I'm not going to get into detail, but suffice to say . . . my showers got much longer after that. And not a single person, including my mother, said anything about it. And there was no shame, no embarrassment, nothing—just a very clean, safe, and happy kid.

Though it might cause some debate with philosophers, I can say with confidence that humans are aware of their bodies—I know this because we have what is called kinesthetic awareness. A person's level of kinesthetic awareness—awareness of their body and its position in space—is actually considered a measure of intelligence by some scientists. Kids spend most of their early childhood developing their kinesthetic awareness. They know when their bodies are moving, when their bodies are still, when their bodies are free, when their bodies are controlled—and they often know when their bodies are changing. For *many* children, part of understanding how their body is changing includes exploring their body. Yes, I mean touching themselves.

That might be difficult to hear for folks who were raised thinking that touching their own bodies was a bad thing, and I recognize how hard this can be to talk about, especially when you're talking about it with your own kids. It might be tempting to put it off, to say *This is something I can talk to them about when they're in puberty and they're actually touching themselves.* The thing is, kids start touching their bodies when they're infants, and often do not stop. How many times have you had to shoo an exploratory hand out of a wet or poopy diaper? Probably more times than you want to reflect on. It's likely that many of you reading this book have a child who uses their arms *and legs* to hug a stuffed animal especially tight as they're falling asleep. No, the fact is that at some point, kids are going to touch their bodies. Providing guidance for our children as they venture into learning about their bodies is part of our jobs as parents. This guidance not only includes making sure their bodies are safe, but making sure their hearts and minds are safe, too.

Figuring out those rules and how to help our children protect their brains requires a healthy dose of education and self-reflection. For many folks, the first step is having to recognize that self-stimulation and body exploration aren't necessarily sexual in the way they've been taught to understand it. There are several proposed reasons why early- and middle childhood-age children self-stimulate. The first is that it is used as a regulatory mechanism—they may rub up against their stuffed animals, touch themselves through blankets, or gravitate toward stuffed toys that vibrate and soothe. Even though that stimulation is technically occurring on their sexual organs, it's not for the type of sexual pleasure that older people seek. Instead, they are using it as a tool to help regulate their central nervous system, calm themselves down, and feel good. Even if a child knows how to deep breathe, meditate, or use mindful movement, self-stimulation is sometimes the best tool for them in the moment, and that is okay.*

Part of helping our children grow up to have respect for their bodies and understand how to keep themselves safe is creating boundaries and rules around safe self-stimulation. Beginning as soon as self-stimulation is a noticed behavior, messaging must be consistent—there is nothing to be ashamed of when you're curious about your body. "You are not wrong or bad, you are curious," "Exploring your body is normal," and "If you are being safe, it's okay for *you* to touch *your own* body."

Again, I acknowledge how hard it might be to say these things to your child, but keep in mind—a child who knows how their body works, who knows what feels good to their body, and who has been allowed to explore

---

*Though self-stimulation in childhood is generally understood to be developmentally normal, there can be situations where self-stimulation is cause for investigation. Markedly increased frequency, unusual engagement with objects such as attempts at penetration, and explicitly sexual displays even after redirection are all examples where concern is warranted, as they can be indicators of potential sexual abuse or exposure to sexually explicit material.

themselves is less likely to be exploring it with anyone else. If they're touching their bodies, they are less likely to be convinced that anyone else should touch them before they are ready.

It's important to know, though, that most coexploration between same-age peers is *completely developmentally normal*—children are just as curious about their friends' bodies as they are their own. It is not a romantic or inherently sexual act—they are trying to build an understanding of the universality of the human experience. "I have these parts, and they look like yours, but not yours. Huh. Interesting." HOWEVER, any power imbalance, coercion, threats, or manipulation to elicit compliance in coexploration, or any activity directed specifically toward sexual stimulation—such as mimicking sex acts—is not considered developmentally appropriate and should be immediately stopped, redirected, and examined.

It is always worth reminding our children of the boundaries around coexploration: "You should explore your own body right now—your brain isn't ready to explore other people's bodies." This is true not because coexploration with same-age peers is damaging—many experts will tell you it isn't. The reason I employ this phrase is because there are people *outside* our children's age range who can and will exploit a child's natural curiosity in order to harm them.

By teaching our children that their body is for them, no one else, not even their friends, we teach them that they can and should say no, and tell us if requests have been made. Because for most of us, that's what we're trying to prevent: our children becoming unsafe and being sexualized too early.

Sample Scripts

Self-Exploration

For me, the goals for the earliest conversations around self-exploration and stimulation are simple: let kids know that it's okay that they're curious and want to touch their bodies, and let them know that there are boundaries for when and how they are allowed to do that. As kids get older, it's important to continue to remind them of the boundaries, but also let them know that self-exploration is a vital part of protecting themselves as they grow.

Early Language/Diaper Wearers (ages 0 to 3)

"You need to keep your hands out of your diapers, bud. There are germs in there from your poop and pee. Let's go wash your hands."

"No hands in pull-ups! They hold germs on your skin and those germs get on your hands."

Try to remember that this sensory-seeking behavior is normal and isn't something shameful—when you're redirecting the behavior, keep in mind that the *diaper* is where the germs are, and that the child themselves is not dirty. Offering an alternative like "Let's make sure you're all clean before you touch your penis/vulva—wait until after bathtime!" can help shape their understanding in a way that does not damage their self-appraisal but also maintains health and safety.

Preschool/Just Potty-Trained Children (ages 3 to 5)

"Stop sign! If you want to put your hands in your pants, then you need to be in your bedroom or in the bathroom."

"Hey, bud! No touching our swimsuit parts when our friends are over. Please take your hands out of your underwear, then go wash your hands."

"I know that feels good, but you need to be in private if you are going to touch your swimsuit area."

Elementary Children (ages 5+)

As children grow, their personal "neighborhood" starts to expand. No longer are they interacting solely with people whom we have vetted—they are beginning to venture into the broader worlds of school, activities, and friends. With this change comes the need for us to become more detailed in the boundaries our children are entitled to as autonomous bodies. This can be a difficult concept to frame for kids this age because previously, they only needed to rely on our judgment—we called the shots about who was safe to help. While we are still their primary safeguard, we can start to explain to children which other adults can intervene in situations where they may need help. Presenting this as levels of care can be a way to make it more understandable: health or safety help, and hygiene help.

"Isn't school so exciting? It really is. I want you to know who your safe grown-ups are at school—who can help you if you have trouble in the bathroom or if you hurt your private parts. The school nurse can help you if you hurt something or if your body is uncomfortable, and they will make sure to call Dad and let me know what's up. You can also let your teacher know if you have a problem in the bathroom, and he will know how to help."

It is a good idea to check in with your child daily to ask how their day went—"Anything exciting happen today? Has anyone in your class ever had to go to the nurse before?"—and maintain open communication regarding their bodies and boundaries. This includes discussing how their own exploration should be carried out.

"Hey, kiddo, please remember the rules about touching your body—you need to be in your bedroom or in the bathroom, you should only be using your hands to touch your body, and your hands need to be washed before you touch."

"I know you're getting really curious about bodies, but please remember that the body you should be most curious about is your own. Your brain still has a lot of learning and growing to do! The best way for your brain to stay safe is to only explore your own body."

Keep in mind that many, *many* children ignore this advice at least once and ask to see (and sometimes touch) the "parts" of their peers. If you have established open communication with your children, you need to be prepared for admissions of "playing doctor" or "I'll show you mine if you show me yours." Same- and similar-age children expressing curiosity over each other's bodies is age-appropriate behavior and should be gently redirected back to self-exploration in private. How you react to your child's admission of boundary pushing will heavily influence how they feel about being open with you in the future. It is *not* unreasonable to alter privileges and supervision for a child who is demonstrating difficulty making sound decisions.

> "Hey, bud. I noticed when Dayvon was over that you were both in the bathroom at the same time. Remember, only one person in the bathroom at a time—privacy!"

> "When your friends were over last time, you chose to play doctor with no clothes on. We keep clothes on for playdates. This week when your friends are here, you will play in the living room instead of in your bedroom."

In these scenarios, you have reminded them that structure and supervision are required for their safety, and that these are not punitive measures—they are chances to practice making good decisions. You have also reinforced that you are not going to react in a way that makes you scary to approach in the future—you are someone who will help your child make choices that keep them safe. It is important, though, to keep in mind the boundaries of curiosity and exploration. **Repeated instances of exploration even after redirection and/or expression of advanced sexual knowledge should be investigated carefully and documented thoroughly. This may mean reaching out to your child's pediatrician, mental health professionals, and other supportive services. If the child is not yours, you may need to reach out to your local reporting agency like Children and Family Services or local law enforcement for investigation and support.**

Middle Childhood (8+)
Why does rubbing your vulva feel good?

> "I want you to think about how good your fingertips are at feeling different things—they can tell hot and cold, they can feel for pressure, they can feel things as soft or hard . . . all kinds of cool skills, right? That's because your fingertips have a lot of nerve endings in them that send signals to your brain and tell your body to feel what your fingers are touching. Your vulva and vagina and all of your muscles around them have some powerful nerves in them, too. Those nerves can feel things like hot and cold and pressure, and they help you know when you need to pee and poop and can send messages to your brain about your body experiencing touch that feels good."

Why does rubbing your penis feel good?

> "Your penis has a lot of nerves in it, just like lots of other places in your body, like your feet. When you rub your penis, your brain makes a chemical called oxytocin that sends a message to your body that makes you feel happy and comfortable. Some people also touch their penis through their clothes because it helps them feel safe and secure."

Adolescents (ages 10+)

Kids in this age bracket are likely to be just a bit more skittish about the topic than their younger counterparts. By this age, most of them have a firmly established sense of privacy that may extend to discussing their bodies. While it is still incredibly important to maintain consent for knowledge, some of these topics may require statements rather than conversations (at least initially) because the information is too important to miss.

For People with a Penis

This next sample script almost broke the internet when I proposed it, but the logic is straightforward. Male condoms are one of the most effective and more accessible forms of STI protection and contraception available; they must be worn by the person with a penis; and (anecdotally) one of the main gripes about them is that sex with a condom "doesn't feel as good." If that is true, and it's also true that using condoms keeps people safe, then it makes sense to encourage young people with a penis to get used to the feeling of wearing a condom, rather than avoid them. And a reasonable, logical time to get used to the feeling of wearing a condom is while self-stimulating.

> "I wanted to let you know there is a box of condoms under the bathroom sink for you. It's really important that you get used to how condoms feel, because they're one of the best ways to protect yourself when you get older and start having sex with a partner. I have one here and I will show you how it works. If you choose to use the condoms while you explore, it might help you get used to the feeling and can also help you not have to clean up as much after you're done. I won't ask you about them or where they are going, but I will check the box every so often and refill them for you. If you want to know more about how they work or if you'd like me to get a different kind, you can always ask me or leave me a note."

"Hey, kiddo. I know we've talked before about you exploring your body, and you know that it's important for you to explore your body before you share your body with anyone else. As you explore, you'll have some cleaning up to do—please clean up after yourself. Tissues are an okay way to clean up, but that can get pretty wasteful. The easiest place to explore and keep clean is the shower."

"As you start exploring, please remember that your penis skin is delicate and can get sore—if it is rubbed too much without anything to protect it, that can cause irritation called chafing. In order to protect it, consider being in the shower or using a lubricated condom. There is also a bottle of water-based lubricant in the bathroom closet that is only for you. I don't care if you use it to lubricate the ball bearings on your desk drawers—if it's gone, I will replace it. If you do find yourself sore or chafed, please either let me know or use the unscented lotion to keep it soothed while it heals. If the unscented stuff stings or you're not getting better, then I need you to let me know so you can get the right kind of cream to help."

"Thank you for letting me know you need more condoms. No, I'm not going to ask you why you need more, I'm just going to ask if you need me to get the same kind or a different kind. Okay, I'll get that kind for you this time. Do you have any questions?"

"Hey, dude, just a reminder—the condoms under the sink are for *you*. Your friends might ask about them and you might be tempted to take some and show your friends, but you gotta remember that not all families are as open with information as we are. If you choose to take one and show your friends, please do not share where we keep them or that you have access to them when you need them. If your friends need access, that's something they need to approach their safe adults to get."

For People with a Vulva/Vagina (ages 10 to 13)

I will never forget the first time the "cucumber" rumor went around my school. Some poor girl in my class (we'll call her Kayla) had made her frenemy angry, and the other girl decided to tell everyone that Kayla had "done it" with a vegetable. All anyone could talk about was how gross she was, how only "sluts" needed to "do it" anyway, and how none of the *normal* girls would *ever* do that—never mind that all of the kids had biological urges to explore their bodies. Kayla was mortified and missed almost a week of school—by that point, the message was clear: Girls don't touch themselves. Media representations of female pleasure still aren't great, so there's work to be done in our homes to help prevent the next generation of kids from experiencing similar shame about their body curiosity.

"Hi, sunshine. I know we've talked before about you exploring your body and understanding how it works before you share it with anyone else. There are a lot of jokes about how people with a penis touch their bodies a lot, but there's not a lot of representation of how people with a vulva touch their bodies. I want you to know that it's totally okay to explore your body and find out what feels good to you. To start, please remember that the best way to explore your body is with your hands and nothing else. Your body is still developing, and until your body is mature it's safest to only rub or touch your vulva, not explore your vagina. Your vagina is growing, just like the rest of your body, so giving it time to finish growing is the best plan before anything goes into it. You don't want to accidentally hurt yourself or end up with an uncomfortable infection."

"I wanted to let you know why it's important to only touch your vulva with clean hands. Your vagina is a self-cleaning system, that's true. If you forget to wash your hands before exploring your vulva, you can end up with an infection, which could be painful or itchy and annoying. So just remember to wash your hands before you touch your vulva. If you *do* end up with a yeast infection or think you might have one, just let me know and we'll get some medication to get it sorted out."

"When your body is sexually excited, it usually makes its own lubricant—it's secreted by these two little glands near the entrance to your vagina. Some people refer to it as 'getting wet.' If your body isn't making that lubricant or isn't making enough of it, or if you're exploring and your body isn't really excited yet, you can use some water-based lubricant. There is a bottle in the bathroom cupboard just for you—no one else will touch it. I don't care if you use it to lube your skateboard wheels—if I notice it's gone, I'll replace it. I just want you to know it's there because if you rub your vulva without lubrication you can end up sore and chafed."

"Hey, kid—I wanted to let you know that part of self-exploration is cleaning up afterward. Whether you rely on the lubrication your body makes or use the store-bought stuff, it's always a good idea to go to the bathroom when you're done exploring. Generally speaking, you should try to pee and then wipe well. This can help you avoid things like urinary tract infections and yeast infections."

"When you're exploring, you will find what feels good to your body—most of that will happen when you are touching and rubbing the outside of your vulva. You might have what's called an orgasm, and that usually involves a lot of the muscles in your pelvic area squeezing and relaxing in waves. You do not *need* to have penetrative sex in order to have one—that is a myth. And maybe it might be a while before you have one—you are not broken if it doesn't happen."

Reminders for Kids Ages 16+

Remember that conversations about bodies don't necessarily stop when a kid grows up. Older kids may need reminders that there are safe and unsafe ways to explore their bodies. By this age, they may have heard about people using things that are shaped like a penis to help people with a vagina explore their bodies. It's important for everyone to know that any internal exploration needs to be done only with items designed for that purpose, like dildos. Kids may also need a reminder to listen to their body—if it hurts, you need to stop.

As I mentioned before, media representation of female pleasure isn't always the best. A pervasive idea I've seen in counseling sessions is that people with a vagina need penetration to reach climax, which isn't true. Dispelling this rumor with my kids is one of the more empowering and protective things I can do for their sexual health, because it puts them firmly in the driver's seat of their own experiences and lets them know they do not need anyone else in order to feel pleasure.

> "It's important to understand that your body does not *need* outside help from a partner or a device in order to feel good. Partners and devices can be part of a healthy sexual life, but they are not *required*. Part of the reason it's important for you to understand how your body works when you are by yourself is because it will help you determine what your boundaries and needs are when you eventually decide you're ready to interact with other people and things."

Explaining Self-Stimulation to a Child with Different Body Parts Than Yours (ages 13+)

Of course, sometimes children grow up in families where only a caregiver with different body parts can provide information about self-stimulation. I think the scripts I've provided above still hold up in this case. Really, the only necessary changes will be to make extra certain that you present the information neutrally—in other words, without judgment and as accurately as possible. For example, you could tell a teen that it's normal for *all* teens to explore their bodies—parts are irrelevant—and that the same rules apply across the board: in private, with clean hands. You can instill in the child that this exploration is not restricted by sex or gender, and that the primary purpose of self-stimulation and exploration is to keep kids safe: safe in their knowledge of themselves, and safe in future situations.

As a reminder, if a child who is not your own asks you questions about self-exploration or self-stimulation, your first answer should generally be "That's a question for your safe adult."

Something's Not Right (all ages)

As adults, we know that there are a myriad of things that can go a little wonky with our bodies. From yeast infections to UTIs to frequent urination, it's hard to keep track of all the things that might end up going a bit sideways. This holds true for children, too. Our kids may need to be encouraged to seek help when things seem "off," especially because they may worry that they did something to cause the change and feel shame about admitting it.

> "I want to remind you that if there is *ever* anything that you feel isn't right with your genitals—if you are extra itchy, or things feel strange, or there are fluids and you're wondering if they're normal—please come to me or another safe adult. I do not want you to avoid asking about things because you're embarrassed or worried that you've made a mistake. My biggest priority in life is making sure you are safe and healthy, and making sure you know who you can come to for help is a big part of that. Do you remember who your safe adults are?"

The Importance of Communication

One of the things that many parents have expressed difficulty navigating is how to both define and communicate body boundaries for their young children. Naturally we want our children to be in the safest of hands, always. We interview daycare providers, pediatricians, and anyone else who may be interacting with our kiddos on a regular basis. We make a short list of individuals whom we trust enough to provide primary care when we are not available. Remembering that we have done this due diligence—we have vetted and carefully chosen these people who will care for our children—will help us know that the next step of the boundary discussion is somewhat simple. If the person is caring for your child, they will care for them appropriately—help them wipe if necessary, take care to make sure they are comfortable, and report any injuries or issues to you immediately.

This may feel scary, because we have all heard horror stories of children being mistreated by carers. However, asking our children to establish or maintain their own boundaries when they are very young is both unreasonable and potentially harmful. If a child is experiencing discomfort because they fell and injured their vulva on the playground but has been told that "no one but Mommy can check their privates," they may fail to report the hurt to their primary carer and delay necessary treatment. Children at this age think of their bodies as neutral—their vulva is not much different from their thumb. If they hurt their thumb, they would tell a grown-up, and it should be the same for their private parts, within limits.

The protection that parents can offer children at this age comes instead from careful due diligence when choosing care providers, providing supervision during peer interactions, and having normalizing daily discussions about bodies and the ways they are treated. Think of yourself as an interviewer—make conversation about their body as normal as reporting what they had for lunch.

> "Did you have a good day at daycare? Great! What was for snack? That's wonderful! Did you get to use the big kid potties today, or did you stay in the classroom? Ooooh, big kid potty?! Cool! Did anyone have to help you?"

A routine like this can not only help you stay connected to the daily activities that your child is experiencing, it can also help you spot anything amiss as quickly as possible. Asking your child how they feel about children at school—new kids, anyone they like or dislike, children who have been labeled as "naughty" or "annoying"—sets a precedence of open-ended communication and lets them know you are invested in their life beyond their health and safety. It also allows you to set boundaries with the adults who care for your child and communicate them effectively and quickly.

> "I heard that you had a new helper start today—sounds like she's a lot of fun! I want you to know that I am not comfortable with her helping Jaxon in the bathroom and I would prefer that you take care of doing that when necessary. Thank you!"

> "Marissa tells me that there is a new kid who is 'naughty'—she said that the playground aide called them that? Can you tell me more about them, and help me understand what she's seeing on the playground and in class?"

CHAPTER 5: IN BRIEF

Curiosity about the human body ranges from information seeking to sensory seeking. This self-exploration, also known as masturbation, is regarded as developmentally normal, though it has been highly stigmatized in many cultures. Helping children understand the health and safety boundaries of self-exploration is an important and often intimidating task for parents. However, parents' proactive choices can both keep their children safe and potentially identify children who have been made unsafe. They can accomplish this by having conversations with their own children about self-exploration, and by understanding healthy boundaries.

Key Takeaways

· Guidance around self-exploration should be free of shame, require privacy, and focus on hygienic practices.

· Privacy during self-exploration means boundaries regarding location (often "bedroom or bathroom") as well as boundaries on participants ("you should only explore your own body").

· Hygienic boundaries are designed to encourage cleanliness and minimize health risks like infection. This includes the "only with your hands" guidance, as well as suggesting individuals with penises explore in the shower or with condoms.

· Providing safe and accurate information to children regarding healthy self-exploration can prevent accidentally dangerous exploration, as well as help protect children from internalized shame that drives poor decision-making and risky behaviors.

CHAPTER 6

Periods, Period.

've said before that I don't have many crystal-clear memories of my childhood—for the most part, there are only a few big moments that stand out as things that I remember. I remember The Talk with my dad. I remember almost lying to my mom about breaking that headband at Claire's. And for some reason, my brain has chosen to remember Period Pancakes.

Fifth grade, when most students are ten or eleven, is when many schools choose to introduce the topic of puberty and sex education. They will send some sort of note home to parents asking if they consent for their child to learn about these topics, and teachers walk the students whose parents sign off through whatever curriculum the school board of their district has been deemed appropriate. My school was no different—fifth grade meant *cue ominous music* sex ed.

This didn't feel like it was going to be a big deal for me—after all, I had already gotten my period. I hadn't *told* anyone that I had gotten my period, but I had what is called "precocious puberty"—in other words, my period started a bit earlier than anyone expected, when I was ten. I had been having regular periods for months at this point, so when my mom said I was going to a class to learn about periods, I figured it would probably be boring, but I'd survive.

Nothing could have prepared me for what that class actually was.

As you might have guessed, we were first split up by assigned gender—girls with Mrs. H and another lady whose name I never learned from some organization in town I didn't bother to register, and boys with Mr. J and his counterpart. Then we were ushered into a room where we were given slips of paper and told to write down questions as they came up. We could pass the slips of paper up at the end and have our questions answered. Everything went downhill after that.

"Hi, girls!" said the lady whose name I never learned. "As Mrs. H said, I'm here to talk to you about puberty and periods. Who here knows what a period is?"

Cautiously, a few of us raised our hands. There was safety in numbers.

"Okay, great! Maybe a few of you know because you have already had your period. Has anyone here already had their period?"

I didn't even need to glance around the room to know there wasn't a soul who was going to raise their hand and risk being the only one. A quick scan told me that I was right to have kept my hand down.

"Oh well, I suppose you all are a bit young, being fifth graders."

Dear God, please don't let anyone see me blushing. She had just told me I was too young to have the thing I had been having for months. I don't remember even a second of the rest of her spiel—my mind was racing, imagining what everyone would think if they knew I already had my period. I sat in this thought spiral as the instructor passed around a model uterus and ovaries and handed out sample maxi pads. She may have talked about how to keep bodies clean, or put a pad into your underwear . . . I honestly don't know. What I do know is that after a few agonizing minutes, she dimmed the lights to show a movie.

The film depicted a fictitious set of friends about our age who are planning a sleepover. Everyone is excited to stay up late talking, laughing, and playing games. During the night, one of the girls wakes up in pain and notices blood on her underwear. The adults in the film discreetly take care of the mess and provide her with the products she needs. The next morning, however, the girls are given a pancake breakfast made by the host's mom. She stands in the kitchen pouring batter on the griddle . . . in the shape of a uterus and ovaries. She's standing there on the screen, using the fluffy breakfast food to explain the menstrual cycle to *her daughter's friend*, as my classmates and I watched in horror.

She gets her period and someone who *isn't even her own mom* explains it with . . . pancakes? In front of her *FRIENDS*? All the questions we'd scribbled on our bits of paper were abandoned—we all wanted class to be done as quickly as possible so we could debrief about the period pancakes. It was the only part of the entire lesson that any of us talked about for days afterward.

I am so grateful that my own curiosity (thanks again, *World Book Encyclopedia*) and my mother's scientific approach to parenting had prepared me for that class. I didn't leave the class in the same state as some of my peers—somehow more confused than they were before and fearing that if they got their period during a sleepover, there might be Menstruation Muffins the next morning.

No, my mom is one of the primary reasons I have approached periods with my own children the way I have. I know that children *all* come from someone who had a period. I know that *many* children will see menstruation at some point, whether depicted onscreen, in a book they're reading, or in their own home. And roughly half of all children will eventually experience a period themselves. Rather than the mysterious blue liquid poured out of a test tube in an ad, or the old adage about a dubious "change" that will some-how "make them a woman" overnight, it's important that we treat periods as what they are: a biological mechanism that is part of the reproductive cycle in people with a uterus. No more. No less.

Treating menstruation this way—matter-of-factly and with only as much fanfare as the child demands—can help prevent children from developing feelings of fear and shame. Instead of "I don't want to bleed to death" or "I hid my bloody underwear for months because I couldn't tell my dad I had my period," let's aim to have children who understand what is happening in their body and who feel capable to obtain the products and information they need to be comfortable at all stages in their cycle.

It's important to know, too, that all this information can and should be given to children who do not have a uterus. They will eventually interact with people who *do* have a uterus—perhaps siblings, friends, or future partners—so it is important that they are equipped with the basic biological facts at the very least.

Sample Scripts

The Vagina is a Self-Cleaning Organ

Early and Middle Childhood (ages 3 to 11)

"Hey, buddy—you're doing a great job of wiping when you go potty! Remember—you gotta wipe from the front to the back. You don't want to get any poop on your vulva!"

"You are learning how to clean your body by yourself and that's really great! When you clean your vulva, I want you to remember that you need to use just a little bit of soap and water on your washcloth and then gently wash your vulva, going from the front toward the back."

Adolescence (ages 12+)

"Now that you have your period, you might think you have to clean your vagina a different way. That is *not* true. Your vagina does not need soap or water or anything else in it to keep it clean. Keep wiping from front to back and ignore any ads you see about 'balancing your pH' or keeping you 'fresh'— you don't need any of those products to keep yourself healthy."

"Please remember that your vagina keeps itself clean—yes, even when you are on your period. You don't need to do anything special *inside* your vagina to 'keep clean.' All you need to be doing is rinsing your vulva with warm water every day, and wiping from front to back after you go to the bathroom."

"You might notice that your vulva has an odor, especially if you have exercised a lot or gotten really hot or sweaty. That smell is from the *outside* of your body—not from your vagina. Clean your body like you usually do, and the smell will go away."

How Do Periods Work?

Early Childhood (ages 3 to 6)

"Mommy is okay—this blood doesn't mean I'm hurt. I am having my period. Every month, my uterus—the place where you grew when you were in my body—pretends it's going to have another baby! It puts tissues on the walls like it's decorating for a baby that might grow there. But when no baby ends up in my uterus, it takes all the tissues down and they come out of my vagina. Then it does it again the next month, just in case I decide I want to have a baby in there."

Middle Childhood (ages 7 to 10)

"You are getting closer to the age where you will probably start your period. You remember that a period is when the uterus grows some additional nutrient-rich tissue inside it just in case the person decides they want to have a baby, right? Well, that tissue, along with some blood, is what comes out of the vagina when a person is having their period. Often for your first period, the blood and tissue doesn't look red like you might expect—they can look brown. Some kids have said that when they wiped during their first period, they thought that their period was poop and that they had wiped incorrectly. But it wasn't poop—it was just the tissue from their first period, so they got some products to help keep their clothes and body clean, and they went about their day."

Adolescence (ages 11+)

"We've talked before about how having a period or menstrual cycle means your body is preparing itself to potentially become pregnant. It does that roughly every month by changing your hormones, and those hormones signal your ovaries—where your eggs stored—to release an egg and your uterus to make itself ready just in case you get pregnant. The lining of your uterus is called endometrium, and it gets thicker and makes a place for the egg to implant if it's fertilized in your fallopian tube. If the egg reaches the uterus and it isn't fertilized (and even sometimes when it is), your body will shed the extra endometrium and the egg—that shedding is your period."

"The average length of a cycle is anywhere from around 21 to around 35 days, and you are most fertile for pregnancy during ovulation, when the egg releases, roughly in the middle of that cycle. It's important to know, though, that you can get pregnant at *any* point in your cycle. A lot of people think that you can only get pregnant when you are ovulating, but since we don't always know exactly when a person is ovulating, it's the safest to assume that you are always at least a little bit fertile."

Discharge

Middle Childhood (ages 8+)

"As you get closer to having your period, you will notice some signs that your body is changing. One of those changes is that your vagina and vulva will start to feel different—there will probably be some fluid that you didn't have before. That fluid is called discharge, and it is completely normal, and can even tell you some important things about how your body is feeling!"

"I choose to wear panty liners in my underwear because I prefer to have the panty liners catch my discharge instead of my underwear. You can wear panty liners if you want, but you do not have to."

"You mentioned that you noticed your underwear changing colors—that is from vaginal discharge. Most people have discharge that is somewhat acidic, and when it comes into contact with the fabric of the underwear, it can bleach the fabric a little bit, making it lighter. If you don't want that to happen to your favorite dark undies, we can get you some panty liners to protect them, if you'd like."

Puberty Prep

Middle Childhood (ages 8 or 9+)

As your child approaches the age where a period is likely to start (as early as age eight or nine, but generally speaking around age eleven or twelve), it is helpful to discuss what to do if their period starts when they are away from home. Consider assembling a Period Preparedness Pack to keep in their bookbag—a spare pair of underwear, a pad, some wipes, and a pair of comfy leggings/shorts that go with anything (I'm a big fan of black leggings for this purpose). This is one of those situations where humor can go a long way toward making upcoming changes feel much more approachable and less scary. Maybe you can give the pack a special or silly name, like "the go bag," "Triple P," "Janitor's Keys," both to remove some of the gravitas of having to pack these items, but also to increase your child's sense of agency and privacy. Only *they* get to decide if they are going to explain why they are carrying an "aisle 7" (as in "cleanup on aisle seven!") in their bag—to everyone else, it's a mystery.

> "Alrighty, let's make sure your school bag is packed and ready! You have your books, pencils, take-home folder . . . Got your aisle seven? Perfect. Sounds like you're all set!"

> "Hey, kiddo—I noticed that you have been saying you're extra tired and that your tummy hurts. You are getting closer to the age where puberty starts, and sometimes before a kid gets their first period they can have some signs to let them know it's coming. Some of those signs include being tired, having cramps, have sore breasts, feeling like your emotions are taking control of your brain, and your hair or skin acting different than you're used to. Remember where the period stuff is, and if you need anything, you can ask me or any of your other safe adults."

Body Odor (ages 9+)

Body odor is another topic that is very charged with people's emotions and morals—we all have thoughts and opinions about how people should or shouldn't smell and what lengths they should go to to meet those ideals. When discussing body odor with kids, it is helpful to highlight their ability to choose their own path and manage their own goals. While we are trying to maintain neutrality about the body—odor is a fact of life—we also must acknowledge that we live in a society where our location and culture will influence how we feel, and how the people around us feel, about odor. The following conversation applies to a child who lives where I live—in the Midwest of the United States—but attitudes may be different where you are:

> "Hey, sunshine—I wanted to let you know that I bought you some deodorant like the stuff I use. I like it because it doesn't have aluminum in it, since there is some evidence that the aluminum isn't good for us, and it helps me feel like the odor my underarms make is not as noticeable as it would be if I didn't use it. You do not *have* to use it, but most of your peers will be using something similar soon if they're not already, and choosing not to use it may be something your classmates comment on. If you want a different kind or a different smell, I'm happy to get it for you."

Emotions (ages 10+)

> "As you go through puberty, you might notice that your emotions feel bigger than they used to—you also might

find yourself saying things impulsively, reacting really fast to things, and just generally feeling stuff way more than you did before. You also might feel like you're at odds with me and other grown-ups. Some of that might be due to your amygdala—part of the emotion center of your brain—growing really fast, and when the amygdala is driving the bus, your thinking brain can't really keep up. I will try my best to remember that this is something you're going through, and I'd really appreciate it if you can try to remember that your amygdala can be a bit of a jerk. We need to be kind and compassionate with each other and try to keep communicating. I might call your amygdala out when it seems like it's taken over—I'll just straight-up say 'AMYGDALA' when you're being a bit much, and that can be our code word for 'let's take a breather and talk once emotions have cleared up a bit.' And you can one thousand percent call me out if I'm chalking things up to your amygdala instead of being a good listener. Sound fair?"

"I also want you to remember that my number one priority is to raise healthy, happy, functional adults. If you are feeling *extra* down—like you can't find pleasure in things you used to love, like you can't enjoy anything, like you don't want to stick around—or just feel shitty in general, I want you to tell me right away so we can get you the support that you deserve. Sound fair?"

Pick Your Products/Product Options

PREPARING FOR A CHILD to start their period takes way more thought than even I realized. There are all the facts that need to be shared about their changing body, all the dry runs of "what to do when it actually happens," and then there are the *products*. Good lord, the products. There are so many options to choose from, and each individual kid is going to have products they like best. The problem, then, is realizing that you have to allow a kid to try multiple things before they settle on what they like best… and that's freaking *expensive*. If you have a child who may someday start a period, I recommend setting aside funds for "product experimentation." Sounds ridiculous to have a savings account just to pay the Pink Tax, but it's a genuine suggestion, especially since some reusable products, such as some period underwear, can cost in the neighborhood of $50.

I've been having my period for over twenty-five years at this point, and and I can still find myself overwhelmed when I walk into the "feminine care aisle." If this is a dizzying experience for an adult, it must be wildly confusing for kids. Thanks to advertising, pads and tampons are fairly well known, but what about menstrual cups? Discs? Period underwear and washable fabric pads? And each of those products has different subtypes, sizes, and absorbancies! How do you even search for what *might* work? To help, here is a quick but inexhaustive rundown of the most common products and some things to consider when picking something for your period novice:

Disposable Pads—absorbent and easy to use by sticking to underwear. Special teen-size pads exist for kids who are smaller/newer to having a period. Pads are often the first period product kids will use. Many pads come with wings to prevent shifting and increase coverage. Pads vary in absorbency from light (panty liners, don't hold much liquid) to overnight (meant to be worn for up to 10 hours and hold a significant amount of liquid). Several different varieties and materials, but all have a limited number of hours that they can be worn before they become unsafe/ineffective and potentially harmful. When they are done being used they should be removed from the underwear and disposed of in the trash. Never flush period products down the toilet, because they can clog the pipes.

Cloth Pads—Very similar to disposable store-bought pads, but washable and reusable. They typically have snaps on the winged parts that help them stay in the underwear. They are made of very absorbent materials like bamboo and have a water-resistant or waterproof backing to protect undergarments and clothes. They can be somewhat expensive and do require special care, but when laundered correctly, they are a cost-effective and eco-friendly alternative to other types of pads.

Tampons—These are typically made of cotton, rayon, or a blend of the two fibers and are made to be inserted into the vagina to absorb menstrual blood. Like pads, they come in many different sizes, absorbencies, and brands. They also come in both nonapplicator types (which must be inserted using your fingers) and varieties with a paper or plastic applicator. Tampons can be particularly helpful during times when the wearer needs to be very active or will be in the water. They can have a steeper learning curve than pads and may require several different tries to find ones that are comfortable and that work. They also must be changed frequently (every 4 to 8 hours), as they carry a risk of complications like toxic shock syndrome (see page 119). Must be disposed of in the trash—never flushed.

Period Underwear—Similar to cloth pads, these are reusable, come in different absorbencies, and require special laundering. Styles vary between brands, and sizing can be tricky. There are usually resources for care and cleaning tips on the manufacturer's website. These can be particularly helpful for individuals with sensory sensitivity to pads and other products, and can be a more positive experience for individuals whose gender doesn't align with "feminine products."

Menstrual Cups—These products are reusable, and come in lots of different sizes and styles, including a wide spectrum of hardness to softness. Menstrual cups are able to hold several hours of menstrual blood, so they're helpful on active days or days spent in the water. Similar to menstrual discs, these cups can take getting used to. The most common complaint, after difficulty finding the correct size, is that they can be difficult to insert—there are numerous different folds and techniques to try. Applicators do exist, but most cups do not come with an applicator. Unlike menstrual discs, cups create a seal with the cervix so removal is done in a specific way so as not to cause pain. Instructions for insertion and removal are generally available with the product and can also be found online. This option can be costly up front, particularly when trying to find the right fit, but once a fit has been found, the product is long-lasting and can save significant funds over time. Care and maintenance usually include washing the cup and sanitizing it occasionally, as well as using wipes. Like other insertable products, these can be associated with complications like toxic shock syndrome or forgotten insertion, though menstrual cups are somewhat more difficult to forget than tampons.

Menstrual Discs—Reusable or disposable depending on the brand, menstrual discs are an insertable device similar to a menstrual cup but flatter. They can be helpful for people with a shortened vaginal canal. They come in different sizes and can take some getting used to; similar to menstrual cups, it can be costly to find the right one. They can hold several hours' worth of menstrual blood, so they can be helpful on very active days or days spent in the water.

Breast Discomfort

Middle Childhood (ages 8 to 9+)

"As you get closer to puberty, your breasts and nipples may get sore as they grow and change. They may also get tender on the days around your period. If you are having some of this discomfort, we can help in a few different ways—by trying different types of bras or different support, using cool compresses, and self-massage. Remember, self-massage should only be in private, and if it's hard to keep yourself comfortable without self-massage, we can find other ways to help you like sweatshirts, camisoles, or bras with some additional padding. You may also notice that your nipples get tender or more sensitive when they get cold. These changes can be really uncomfortable but also really exciting for your body, so we just need to keep checking in and making sure that you are feeling your best."

Once Periods Have Happened, or Conversations for Adolescents

I was watching a lovely television show—*Call the Midwife*—recently, and I was reminded how infrequently people in previous generations discussed body functions, particularly menstruation. I then reflected on my own experience as a young person, and realized that the shroud of mystery and shame, while lessened, definitely still exists. This secrecy was part of what prompted me to identify exactly how I propose talking to older teens about menstruation. My approach requires acknowledging that just because someone has had a period doesn't mean they don't have questions about menstruation or need support.

> "Hey, kiddo, you know a lot about how periods work, but I wanted to remind you that if there's ever anything you think might be wrong, you really should come to me and let me know. Or go to another one of your safe adults, that's okay, too. If you get to fourteen or fifteen and you haven't had your period yet, let me know. Maybe we can get that checked out."

> "Just a reminder—if you have anything that feels weird or off, please tell me. If you're itchy or sore, let me know. There can be lots of things going on, but also you might have a yeast infection. Having a vulva and vagina can be a lot to figure out, and I don't expect you to try to navigate all of this all by yourself. I've done it, and I've been doing it for a lot of years, so I can totally help you understand what might be going on with your body. And I can also help you find help if you need it."

Body and Product FAQs

I don't want to wear tampons because they feel weird and/or hurt. Am I doing something wrong?
It's not a matter of doing something wrong, it's a matter of practice and fit. You're right—your tampon shouldn't hurt. It might be that the angle isn't

quite right—try adjusting the angle that you use to put it in. It may be that you have a shorter vaginal canal and either need to use a smaller product or to adjust the tampon to sit so it's not poking your cervix. Either way, you can practice putting them in with a little bit of lubricant and see if you can find a way that is consistently comfortable. And if not, we can find you an alternative!

What do I do if I'm not sure if I left a tampon/disc/cup in?

That can be a medical emergency, so it's important to take a few steps as quickly as you think of it: First, use a finger to see if you can feel the string of your tampon/lip of your disc/stem of your cup. If you can, great! You can pull it out. If you can't find the string/lip/stem and you're still worried you left one in, use a hand mirror to check if you can see anything in your vagina or anything you could grasp for removal. If you can't see anything, then it's probably a good idea for us to make an appointment with your doctor so we can make sure you don't end up with an infection or toxic shock syndrome.

Okay, but what is toxic shock syndrome?

Toxic shock syndrome (TSS) is a rare complication of certain bacterial infections. If a tampon, menstrual disc, or menstrual cup is left in the body for too long *and* has the required bacteria, the body can react to that bacteria and cause TSS. This complication can cause high fever, low blood pressure, and vomiting or diarrhea, and can even be life-threatening. Once an individual has had TSS once, it is more likely they will get it again, and they should not use tampons, discs, or cups anymore.

What do I do if my period hurts like, really, really bad?

If your period hurts, please tell me. There are several things that we need to consider if you are having a painful period. The first is that a certain amount of cramping and discomfort is normal during a period—your body is contracting muscles to help shed the lining of your uterus. We can get you some hot compresses and pain relievers, and increase your activity to help with some of that lower-level discomfort. If you are having very painful periods, however, we need to consult your doctor and have you assessed for other causes like endometriosis. I will help you advocate for the help you need.

Is there ever a time I should be worried about smelling bad?

We've talked before about how your vulva might have an odor, particularly after a lot of exercise or being in hot weather, and that normal cleaning can help manage that smell. If you notice that the smell *doesn't* go away, or that the smell has changed, please let me know so we can head to your doctor. A change in smell is one of the first signs of a bacterial infection, which will need to be treated with medication.

How come my period always surprises me? What the heck, Mom?

Well, kid, sometimes the frequency of your periods can be difficult to pinpoint. There's lots of different reasons for this. Part of it might be that you're just young and your hormones haven't balanced out. It could have to do with your weight fluctuating from season to season (but if your period's not coming because you're too thin, we need to talk to your doctor). Or it could have something to do with other hormonal things like polycystic ovarian syndrome (PCOS). If this irregularity is really bothering you, we'll absolutely make an appointment with your doctor and try to figure out some answers, but for now, we can also just keep track and see if there's a pattern we recognize. Sound fair?

Mom, what does it mean to pop somebody's cherry?

Oh, okay, so. In some people's vaginas, there's this little flap or circle of tissue called the hymen. It's leftover tissue from embryonic development—it's like a little ring or crescent shape just around the opening of the vagina that doesn't serve any purpose that we know of. But the reality is that many people don't have one. When there *is* a hymen, it can be stretched to the point that it bleeds, which some people call "breaking" the hymen. This can happen in lots of different ways—from using a tampon, having a bump or fall that impacts the pelvis, exploring your own body . . . you get the idea. Some folks' hymens are more than just a little ring—it can actually be a thin covering over the opening of the vagina that needs to be surgically corrected to make penetration possible, but that's pretty rare. "Popping someone's cherry" is part of a larger, really damaging myth that if a person with a vagina hasn't had sex before, they will bleed after their first time. Get it? The "cherry" is the blood after someone's hymen breaks? Yeah. But since we know that not everyone even *has* a hymen, and that it doesn't need to "break" . . . Exactly. People might assume that a vagina is "used" if it doesn't bleed after penetration. And if there is really high value placed on sexual purity where that person lives, this myth can be reallllly dangerous.

CHAPTER 6: IN BRIEF

Menstruation has been treated with secrecy and shame in many cultures, but accurate and honest conversations about menstruation are developmentally appropriate beginning in early childhood. A period is, at its core, a biological mechanism that is part of the reproductive cycle. Children may experience many emotions when learning about menstruation ranging from curiosity to fear to disgust, but by normalizing the process, parents can potentially prevent those strong reactions from turning inward and resulting in shame.

Key Takeaways

- The vagina is a self-cleaning organ—it does not need to be cleaned internally with products like douches or with soap, despite advertisements to the contrary.

- Menstruation occurs when the endometrium (lining) of the uterus, which is made of nutrient-rich tissue, is sloughed off and ejected through the vagina. In anticipation of hosting a fertilized egg, the endometrium grows back, but if fertilization does not occur, menstruation begins again. This cycle recurs monthly for some people, and at less predictable intervals for others.

- People with a uterus typically begin menstruating around the same time they are experiencing puberty (though other health factors can impact this), so preparation for periods should start when signs of puberty begin to appear.

- Periods can also coincide with other body changes like increases in vaginal discharge, breast discomfort, body hair, and body odor.

CHAPTER 7

Pen15 Club

"Dude," Jessica said with alarm, "I can see your pubes!"

"What?" her son Mason replied quizzically.

"I can see . . . what are you doing? I can see your pubic hair!"

"Oh, sorry."

"Why are you pulling on the front of your swim trunks like that? I get it, these new swim jammers are way tighter than your normal trunks, but like. What is going on? You need to stop that."

"Uh, no. I won't be stopping that. Thanks," Mason said dismissively.

"Wait, what?" Jessica was shocked, and with her eyebrows that far into her hairline, Mason knew he had to explain.

"I learned at swim team initiation that I can't stop."

"Whoa, whoa, whoa, whoa, whoa. Back the truck up. What do you mean, 'initiation'? WHAT IS GOING ON?!"

"Okay, Mom, don't freak out."

It was too late. Jessica was freaking out. Her son, a seventh grader, had just joined the swim team. He was lanky and lean and actually quite quick in the water. He also loved swimming. The swim jammers were a somewhat new experience for him, though, and much tighter than normal swim trunks. It had taken him a bit to get used to them, and now every time he got out of the pool he was pulling out the front of them, way too close to showing people what was underneath. If he pulled just a little bit farther, there would be nothing left to the imagination. This was not okay, and if the older boys on the team were leading him to do this, she had a really big issue on her hands.

"Mom, let me explain."

"Okay, I told you I'd always listen, so I'm listening."

"I didn't know that with the temperature of the pool and the way that swim jammers work, when I get out of the pool, they kind of like . . . vacuum seal to my penis."

"What?" Jessica asked. This had taken . . . a sharp left turn.

"Yeah, they like, suction on and I didn't know. I was just getting out of the pool, but the older boys showed me what they meant," Mason explained patiently.

"I am still so confused."

"Mooooom. When I get out of the pool, it suctions onto my penis, and you can see every outline of *everything*. How long it is. How big it is. If it's really, really cold, or if it's going to get . . . you know. Do you get my drift?"

"Oh." She did, indeed, get his drift.

"So the older boys told me that when you get out of the pool, if you just pull the top of the waistband a little bit, it like, loosens up and then you can't see as much. I promise I won't pull it out quite as far. I'll try to make sure that you can't see everything," he offered as a sort of compromise.

"My dude, that's totally fine. I understand now. Thank you for telling me. I am sorry I didn't get it before."

"It's okay, Mom. You don't have one and you're not a swimmer, so I don't expect you to know. I didn't."

It can be really hard to talk about the parts you don't have, because you've never lived the experience of having them. If you don't have a penis, you don't know at all what it's like to wake up with "morning wood," and you don't have any idea what it's like to have a surprise erection in the middle of class. If you've never had to navigate it, guiding a child through how to handle it can be intimidating. It might even be tempting to use books or movies or other media to allow the education to happen without you. Supplementing our children's education is exactly what this book is aiming to do, right? But the goal shouldn't be for our children's education about their bodies to happen without us—that's not fair to our children, or to us. No amount of representation or factual written word can replace information presented with love, thoughtfulness, and guidance by their caregivers.

"Mama?" the sweet voice said sleepily from the foot of the bed.

Barely registering her consciousness, much less the small human next to the bed, Marcy replied, "What's up, baby?"

"Something is wrong with my penis."

Well, she was awake now. "What do you mean, something is wrong with your penis? Are you hurt? Did something happen when you tried to go potty?"

"It's . . . long."

Now her brain was on overdrive. She felt like essentially any other adjective would have registered better than "long." But there she was at 6 a.m., trying to figure out what might cause a "long penis."

"Long? What . . . what do you mean?"

"Look at it!!"

What even is life?! Her three-year-old was standing next to her bed, undies around his ankles, concernedly showing her his "long penis."

Time for the erection conversation.

"That's called an erection, sweetheart. It just means that your penis has a lot of blood in it and that makes it look like it's a bit . . . longer. You might notice that it feels stiff or hardened, too. That happens to most people with a penis, and it will go away soon. No need to worry. You can just go potty and go back to bed."

She thought about telling him that erections are normal, or that they happen at night all the time, or that it was a sign his body was working as expected. But it was the middle of the night, they were both exhausted, and the odds that he would internalize anything more than the base message of "Mom gave you science and said to go back to bed" were slim. So she decided that she'd already said more than technically necessary, turned back over, and fell asleep.

Or tried to. A few moments later, after almost dozing off, she heard a frustrated groan from the bathroom. As she crossed the threshold into the bathroom, she spotted a poor little kid who had not accounted for physics. There was pee pretty much everywhere—the floor, his jammies, the shower curtain—and he was holding his still erect penis down in the toilet bowl. He had forgotten to aim. As he locked eyes with her, he spouted wisdom that can only come from the lived experience of having a penis:

"Sometimes these things just don't behave."

Explaining exactly how "these things" work is probably a whole lot easier when you have your own experience to fall back on. Much like someone with a uterus can't perfectly convey what it's like to experience menstrual cramps, I am certain that no description of being "kicked in the balls" has ever captured what it actually feels like. The thing is, though, even when I describe my menstrual cramps to another person with a uterus, they won't ever know if what I'm describing is exactly what they feel because they can't be inside my body, feeling what I feel. This is the reason I remind parents that they need to listen as much as they talk, even if it's about a common experience. Similarly, that listening has to come from a safe, nonjudgmental viewpoint—kids need space to share their perspective, especially if it differs from the "norm," and they need support. In my experience, the quickest way to shut a child down and leave them feeling like they have to go it alone is to make it seem like you're going to judge them.

I'd be lying if I told you we can't leave kids to figure stuff out on their own—it's an option! The internet exists, and even if we skip giving our kids the "this is how you research" talk, they'll get at least a few bits of accurate information, all things considered. However, if we want our kids to have accurate information that will keep them safe, healthy, and happy, we *must* be involved in the discussions, at least somewhat. So if we feel unsure, then it's up to us to take the first step in handling these conversations about body parts—the ones we have and the ones we don't: educating ourselves. In chapter 6, we got a crash course in what kids need to know about having a period, as well as other body changes that happen during puberty. This chapter covers similar topics, but also addresses some of the stereotypes that often accompany the physical changes of puberty for young people with a penis. Because ultimately, changing bodies can be confusing and disorienting, especially when the information you're getting from outside sources doesn't match the information you've been raised with.

Sample Scripts

What Is An Erection?

Early Childhood (ages 2 to 6)

"Your penis/the baby's penis is long and feels/looks stiff like that because it has extra blood in it right now. That happens sometimes! It will stop eventually."

"I know it feels different when your penis has an erection, and you can touch it if you want, but only in your bedroom or in the bathroom, by yourself, and with clean hands."

Middle Childhood (ages 7 to 10)

"Erections—when the penis gets full of blood so it looks longer and feels harder—happen for lots of different reasons and at lots of different times. Sometimes people wake up with an erection, sometimes they have them when they are excited about another person, and sometimes they happen for no real reason at all. Eventually they go away on their own, but sometimes people choose to touch their erection for a while because it feels good, and then it goes away."

Adolescence (ages 10+)

Helping a child navigate their changing body is always going to include helping them deal with potentially embarrassing situations (I was pretty sure I would never live down my pad leaking through my jeans at youth group). For people with a penis, this means preparing them for the sneak-attack erections that can happen as they go through puberty (and beyond). This includes not only warning them they might experience these sneak attacks and helping them figure out how they can build "concealment systems" into their everyday lives, but also reminding them that they are *not* alone.

> "You may have erections at the most random times—they might happen when you expect them to, like after seeing an attractive person, but they can also happen after things that you never expected. Getting an erection does *not* say anything about what you like or what's happening in your brain. All it means is that your body decided now was a good time to fill your penis with blood. As you get through puberty, the erections will calm down some and happen at less annoying, more predictable times."

> "If you are worried about getting an erection during school, you might want to consider getting a binder that you can keep your notebook and pen in and use as a cover. You can also wear thicker pants like jeans or sweats, or carry a sweatshirt with you. You have options."

"I'm going to share with you one of the best things I ever heard, from my friend Warren when we were sixteen. He told me there's really no reason to bother worrying about covering up a sneak-attack erection because at your age, they're happening to everyone. Just try not to stare at anyone else's, wait it out, don't be a jerk when it happens to other people, and you'll be fine. You're all in the trenches together on this one."

Nocturnal Emissions (Wet Dreams)

Middle Childhood/Adolescence (ages 8 or 9+)

"Pretty soon you may start to have erections while you're sleeping—you may have already woken up with an erection. As you get older, this might happen more, and you may notice that sometimes you wake up and your underwear feels damp or wet. This means that your body ejaculated—released some semen from your penis—while you were asleep. Semen is the liquid that carries sperm cells out of your testicles—it's *not* pee. This is totally normal and something that most people with a penis experience. When it happens, you should clean yourself off with a damp cloth or a wipe and put your underwear in the hamper or in the washing machine. Please make sure you fold it in a way that no one will accidentally touch the semen if they are doing the laundry."

Body Hair

Early and Middle Childhood (ages 3 to 11)

Again, facts and neutrality are the approach for children at this age.

"The hair that's on swimsuit parts is called pubic hair. It grows there for lots of different reasons. People grow it when they get older—most kids your age don't have it. Some grown-ups choose to remove their pubic hair, but everyone gets to pick what works best for them."

Shaving

Adolescence (ages 12+)

"I wanted to let you know that I bought shaving cream, some aftershave, and a razor for you and left them in the bathroom. You don't have to use them yet, but you might want to consider starting to experiment with them. I do not expect you to shave right now because you're not really growing much on your face, but eventually you'll probably want to learn how to because it's a fun way to play with how you look. You know Grandpa has a beard, but Uncle Tony has a goatee. And lots of folks, you know, just have bare faces. It's just a fun form of self-expression. Just make sure you use the shaving cream, and you shave along with the direction of your hair. I can show you how to do it, or we can find some videos online if you'd like."

Body Odor

Middle Childhood (ages 10+)

"Hey, dude—check your dresser. I left a couple sticks of deodorant on top. You don't technically have to wear deodorant, but we live in a part of the world where folks expect people to have pleasant body odor, or at least neutral or no body odor. Most people don't have that naturally, so I bought you some different deodorant scents. They're kind of like cologne—you can pick which one you like or smells the best to you, or just go with the one that has the least scent—it's up to you! I also want to remind you that you need to be taking showers every day. Or at least every other day. That's important for helping to control body odor, but it's also important to help keep your body clean and healthy."

Physical Changes (Muscles, Height, Voice)

Middle Childhood (ages 8+)

"I noticed that everybody in your class is starting to become all different heights. Isn't that wild? Yeah, some of you are getting closer to puberty, which means your bodies are going to start changing a lot. I want you to remember that you can always come to me with questions, and even though I don't have the same parts as you, I can either tell you the answer or help you find the answer somewhere else."

"Hey, kiddo, you're getting to an age where people are going to be changing a lot and at very different rates. Some people are going to get tall really fast, whereas others are going to take longer to grow and not get as tall. Some people are going to really bulk out, they're going to get a lot of muscles super fast, and other people are going to stay like a string bean. Some people, like us, are going to put on a little bit of extra weight to help fuel getting taller and more muscular. All these changes can feel really awkward, especially because it feels like most people aren't changing at the same rate as you. The truth is, they're not, and that's okay."

Self-Exploration—Again

If you're reading this book straight through, you might be wondering why the following scripts seem like a reiteration of chapter 5. The reason stems from both my professional experience and the anecdotal experiences of other professionals. Children may be feeling lots of increased curiosity during this time in their lives. They want to explore their bodies because they know it feels good. This may lead to an uptick in frequency of self-stimulation, but the co-occurring onset of puberty can also mean an uptick in shame and secrecy. I think about the language surrounding teen masturbation in books, movies, and television shows: "jerking it," "stiff socks," "crispy towels," served with a heavy side-eye and jabs about being horny, but very little acknowledgment of what might actually be the most comfortable and safe. The following scripts are just slightly different from the ones found in chapter 5 and are meant to help you, the caregiver, reiterate important information without feeling like a broken record.

"We've talked before about how it's totally normal for you to want to explore your body. That's just as true now as it has ever been, but now that you're getting older, you might feel like you want to do that more often. That's *also* okay."

"As you get older and your body changes, you might stimulate your penis enough to have what's called an orgasm. That's where your body ejaculates semen—it's how you release the sperm cells needed to make a baby. It adds an extra step of cleanup to the process, so you have to be a little bit thoughtful about where you're doing that. The shower is a good option because it essentially takes care of cleanup for you."

"Hey, bud—I don't super care how long your showers are, but please remember to stick with just water if you're going to be touching yourself. Shampoo, conditioner, and soap can all irritate your urethra and give you an infection, so let's skip that."

"As a reminder, there's a box of condoms under the sink. You do not have to use them. They are there for you whenever you need to use them. I would encourage you to maybe consider using them if you're gonna explore yourself because it's a great way to get used to the feeling of wearing one. They're going to be necessary when you become sexually active with whoever you become sexually active with, so . . . use them. Make sure you throw them away in the garbage can underneath the sink. If you need a refill, let me know, or I'll just try to keep an eye on them and replace them when they're running low. They're for you."

"I found my bottle of fancy lotion when I was cleaning your room. I'm not mad that you used it, but I swapped it out for the unscented stuff from the bathroom because I don't want you to end up possibly uncomfortable."

Masculinity

In my own life I've found that if I were to ask ten people what it means to be masculine, I would very likely get ten different answers. There have been countless books, podcasts, op-eds, and articles written about the right way to "be a man." The stereotype that has spurred a huge portion of this discourse is that men can either be happy and horny or angry and aggressive. The confusing part for people growing up identifying as men is that those books, podcasts, op-eds, and articles don't all agree with the scientific results that tell us this binary is patently false. Frustratingly, not only are some of the voices in the discussion screaming that the binary is true, those voices are also the most easily accessible. Thankfully, there *are* credible resources, and I've shared them with you on page 285 to help you shape the conversations about masculinity you have with your child. But in the meantime, here are some sample scripts to help you help your child navigate what it means to be a man.

Emotions (ages 10+)

"As you go through puberty, you might notice that your emotions feel bigger than they used to—you also might find yourself saying things impulsively, reacting really fast to things, and just generally feeling stuff way more than you did before. You also might feel like you're at odds with me and other grown-ups.

Some of that might be due to your amygdala growing really fast—it's part of the emotion center of your brain, and when it's driving the bus, your thinking brain can't really keep up. I will try my best to remember that this is something you're going through, and I'd really appreciate it if you tried to remember that your amygdala can be a bit of a jerk. We need to be kind and compassionate with each other, and we need to try to keep communicating. I might call your amygdala out when it seems like it's taken over—I'll just straight up say 'AMYGDALA' when you're being a bit much, and that can be our code word for 'let's take a breather and talk once emotions have cleared up a bit.' And you can one thousand percent call me out if I'm chalking things up to your amygdala instead of being a good listener. Sound fair?"

"Uh, dude, I want to make sure we're on the same page—that movie that said people need to 'man up' and 'stop being a . . . derogatory word for female genitalia'? That movie was from my childhood. It's *not* a healthy representation of what it means to be a man. People with a penis feel just as many emotions as people who don't have them, and the idea that identifying as a man somehow means you suddenly have only two settings—horny and angry—is stupid. You have always done a great job of talking about your feelings—that doesn't have to change just because you're growing up into a man."

"I also want you to remember that my number one priority is to raise healthy, happy, functional adults. If you are feeling *extra* down—like you can't find pleasure in things you used to love, like you can't enjoy anything, like you don't want to stick around—or just feel crappy in general, I want you to tell me right away so we can get you the support that you deserve. Sound fair?"

"I was thinking about what you said the other day—how you think you don't 'feel' as much as other people, and they don't seem to like it. I'm not positive that I'm interpreting what you meant correctly, but it sounds to me like you're saying that other folks get really *big* emotions, and they express them a lot, and you don't really do that. And they think that means you don't care, even when you do. Are you worried about your feelings, or are you worried about how people perceive you? Either way, you are not broken or wrong simply because you experience and react to the world differently. Emotional skills are something all people have to learn and work on—no one comes out of the womb knowing that stuff!"

I remember being a teenager and watching the way television and movies talked about teen boys. Entirely too often, the underlying message was that all they wanted to do was "get some." I can think of a laundry list of stories where being sexually active very early and very often was a driving plot point for the male characters. I also remember that characters who expressed their emotions or who were vocal about their feelings were treated as "soft" or "girly"—that in order to solidify their place in the high school pecking order, they had to abandon their emotional inner self in favor of being a tough, sexually active, popular guy. I also remember making the conscious decision to raise my own children very differently. I never wanted my child to feel like they had to determine where they fit in the hierarchy of high school popularity by compromising their own feelings or values.

> "You do not have to change who you are or what you want for your own body just to fit in. People who are bragging about their sexual conquests are jerks who do not respect their partners and are quite possibly lying. You do what *you* feel ready for, and you don't go broadcasting what you *do* choose to do for clout. Got it?"

Big Kids Still Want to Play

Something we forget is that when children, particularly male-identified children, grow up, they still want to participate in play. The hard part, I think, for kids who are going through puberty in the United States is the more recent cultural expectation that they shift from play to organized sport. Encouraging and facilitating non-sports play is one way to foster their social and emotional development as they enter puberty. Try yard games like bean bags, bocce, or spikeball; field games; or unstructured physical activity like tag, (boundaried) roughhousing/wrestling, even pool noodle sword fights. Be creative!

If Something Might Be Wrong

> "Hey, kiddo—I just wanted to remind you that if you *ever* have problems with any of your parts—if something is sore, or itchy, or just feels 'off'—you can come to me and we'll find you appropriate help, okay? Even if you think it's happening because of something you did or a mistake you made—all I care about is that you are safe and healthy. Please come to me if you need help."

CHAPTER 7: IN BRIEF

Changing bodies can be incredibly confusing, disorienting, and sometimes downright scary. For people with a penis, changes (like erections) sometimes occur with an element of surprise that can add a layer of shame and embarrassment to the process. Children who have been informed of the scientific facts about these changes, and who have been given accurate information and space to ask questions, may feel more empowered to navigate the changes and potentially feel less stress than if they had been left to figure things out on their own via trial and error.

Key Takeaways

- Erections occur when the brain sends messages to the body instructing it to fill the penis with blood. Erections are not necessarily indicative of sexual attraction—they *can* be, but they can also occur spontaneously.

- Body changes for people with a penis are not dissimilar from the changes that occur for people with a uterus—they include changes in height, voice, musculature, body hair, body odor, and more.

- Additionally, children may experience an additional drive for self-stimulating behaviors, and should be provided with safe, healthy, sanitary options for managing these behaviors.

- One such option is encouraging condom use while self-stimulating, which theoretically could lead to increased ease of use, and may lead to more consistent use of condoms in future sexual relationships.

CHAPTER 8

Where Do Babies Come From?!

This is it. This is the chapter I know most of you are reading this book for. You might've picked this book up off the shelf and flipped directly to this chapter because you want to just get it over with—you want to prepare yourself for the conversation you've been dreading. But first, take a deep breath and remember that this is the chapter where a lot of us are going to have to go back and do the internal work of processing the trauma and embarrassment we internalized when we were given the "birds and the bees" talk.

The "you're going to have sex, get pregnant, or get a disease and die" talks.

The "why buy the cow when you can get the milk for free" talks.

The "no one likes a used piece of gum," "no one wants a pre-licked lollipop," and "no husband/wife wants damaged goods" talks.

Purity culture, fearmongering and misunderstanding around sexually transmitted diseases, and the specter of a life-altering unplanned pregnancy too often guide discussions around sex and intimacy as children are growing up. Regardless of where your morals are regarding when sex should happen, we can *all* agree that if people are going to have sex, they should have it in the safest way possible. A lot of us parents now know that we must be willing to have more nuanced, open, honest conversations with our kids if we want to both keep them safe and help them feel empowered to have the best relationships they can. That is why, if you did flip directly to this chapter, I encourage you to go back and read the first section of this book, "Foundations" (page 14). It will help set you up for predominantly positive outcomes from these tough conversations by solidifying the safe, loving groundwork you've laid with your child. Two of these Foundations, Curiosity and Consent for Knowledge, guided me through explaining my first nephew to my own child.

"There's a BABY in there!" I pointed enthusiastically at my sister's growing belly, letting my child in on the most exciting news I'd heard in a while. "In a few months there's going to be a new baby coming!"

My kid's response was to be expected—he was eighteen months old, so this was all very abstract—so he mirrored my excitement by clapping and giving me a "yay!"

A couple of years later, as my first round of friends started having children, my child got a little bit more invested in this "baby in the tummy" business. The fact that the baby was in there was taken for granted—he knew that was where babies grew—but the questions were getting a bit more existential.

"Mom, where do babies COME from?" he asked me one sunny winter afternoon shortly after his fourth birthday.

"They come from inside a person's uterus!" I replied.

"Ohhhhhh, okay." Satisfied at now knowing the name of the organ where a baby grew, my kid went back to playing. That didn't last long, though.

"How does a uterus make a baby?" was the next question I had to field, just a few weeks later.

"Well, it's super cool! There are two cells—one is called a sperm, and one is called an egg—and they each have half of the instructions needed to make a baby! You know, like your building sets—the instructions say which pieces go where, but each cell only has half! So the cells get together and share instructions with each other, and then the cells multiply and click together like the building pieces and make a baby!"

This. Was. MIND-BLOWING. My child chewed on this information, rehashing it over and over again, for months. It wasn't until a couple of *years* later that I finally got the question I'd been gearing up to answer.

"Mom . . . how do the cells get INTO the uterus to combine?"

You might think this is where our journey to answering "where do babies come from?" really kicks off, but that is not so. Our story begins all the way back when kids first start realizing that there are many humans other than themselves, and that some of those humans are babies. As we journey into answering any questions for our kids, it's essential that we remember the lens through which they view the world—a lens that has only seen a few things and understands even fewer. Our job, then, is to give only the information that answers the question at hand, and in the simplest way possible. This is in line with a theory called scaffolding. Developed by psychologist Lev Vygotsky, it describes how information should be presented in small pieces that build upon previously presented pieces in order to create larger ideas. Many conversations with adolescents would not be as easy, or even possible, if they were not built onto information presented to the child earlier in life.

In order to help build your child's knowledge base, I've broken down "where do babies come from?" into a series of basic steps that scaffold on one another. By following the steps in order, you may be able to avoid overwhelming your child with information they are not ready to understand, process, or internalize. Additionally, by having the information sectioned into smaller pieces, you have the answers to the next suite of questions at hand when your child is ready to hear them!

These conversations are not prescriptive to a certain age range—there is no one right age to have Mechanics conversations with your children—but I have included rough estimates of when a child may feel ready to approach their safe grown-ups with the questions from each section. I arrived at these estimates by combining a few different sources: my own personal and professional experience; the opinions of other child development professionals; and the psychological concepts I've mentioned previously in the book, such as Piaget's theory of cognitive development—plus a concept I haven't previously mentioned called theory of mind.

This theory posits that children do not develop the ability to see other people's perspectives or even acknowledge that other people think differently than they do until they are in the ballpark of four to six years old. This inability to "zoom out" informed the way I wrote the scripts for younger children in this book.

Despite the theoretical lenses that contribute to the age-range recommendations, as we discussed earlier in the Consent for Knowledge chapter, one of the most important people to consult when deciding what information a child is ready for is the person asking the questions—the CHILD! Giving a child information about the content they are requesting gives them a sense of ownership over their knowledge. It also models to them that people's right to choose what they know is of utmost importance—"The answer to that question might make you feel some interesting feelings, and it's something other folks might choose to wait to learn."

As I'm certain you've noticed already, the bulk of the language in this book is meant to be tailored to the child you are currently raising. However, as we venture into the topic of where babies come from, we must eventually discuss with our children the parts that they do not have. This is where we have to talk about the language I choose to use in this book—it is very biological and almost entirely gender-neutral. This might feel very foreign, even somewhat off-putting, but the language used in this discussion matters, and so does the confidence you feel in delivering this information to your child. However, if you are more comfortable using words like "mom" and "dad" or "man" and "woman," that is a valid choice. (Just be prepared for follow-up questions like "What about Tim? He doesn't have a dad?" or "My friend Carly has two moms—where did she come from?!")

Being clear from the outset that the cells we are talking about come from a person with a penis and a person with a vagina, and those cells grow in a uterus, you can build a sense of clarity and honesty that are routinely reinforced with every conversation. Later, as they interact with more children from different backgrounds—adoption, IVF, and other less traditional methods of building a family—being adept with accurate biological terminology will matter even more. There will be no question that although Carly had to grow from cells from a person with a penis *and* a person with a vagina, Carly's moms *are* her moms.

And as we discussed previously, using correct terminology helps children feel comfortable talking about their bodies with universally understood terms.

As children grow, they need to be able to clearly and unashamedly report injuries or other important information about their bodies to their caregivers. A child who has been taught to call their vulva a "cookie" may report to their pre-K teacher that their "cookie is yucky"—and without context, the teacher would have no idea that this child is uncomfortable because they are having trouble wiping when they go to the bathroom. Using clear, accurate words not only keeps our children healthy, it also protects them from people who might wish to harm them and will exploit a child's ignorance and innocence to do so.

As I've said earlier, one of the most important reasons for establishing body talk as a routine part of your child's life is that it can help keep them safe. If your child approaches you with a question that seems premature, consider attempting to find out why the child is asking: "That's an interesting question—what do you think about it?" Asking questions like that can help you parse if they are truly seeking the information you *think* they're seeking, or if there's been a misunderstanding or miscommunication. Further, it can help you determine if your child has access to information they should not have or if they are being exposed to things they are not prepared to see, such as being in the presence of a relative watching movies that are inappropriate for a child their age.

Sometimes it may even be necessary to let your child know that the information they are seeking is not information they are ready to receive: "I understand you're curious about that because you heard it on the podcast your uncle was listening to, but that kind of language and information is for grown-up brains—your brain is still growing and learning, and when it's ready, I promise I'll answer that question for you. We can even write it down so I don't forget." Demonstrating that you are willing to both set and maintain boundaries that help protect their development and maintain their safety reinforces that you are there to help them. It reminds your child that you want them to learn in a way that is healthy, and you want them to have information that will empower them rather than frighten or overwhelm them. These boundaries may also help curb an older child's desire to seek information for themselves from dubious peer resources or the internet.

Sample Scripts: Early Childhood

Phase One: Where Do Babies Grow? (birth to age 3)

This "conversation" isn't so much a sit-down-and-talk conversation as it is a combination of observations and a general way of viewing the world. Establishing curiosity and a desire to make observations about the world we live in is one of the foundational pieces of these body talks. So at this stage of the game, we are mostly just observing and commenting on what we notice about pregnant bodies and the general process of being pregnant, like the number of weeks the baby has been growing or someone needing to sit down more often. Here are some phrases that you might want to include as you and your child notice pregnant people:

"That person has a baby growing in their uterus!"

"Auntie Kay has a baby growing—it will be born in July! That means that we will have Christmas, your birthday, the end of school, and camping before the baby is born."

"That baby is really tiny—I think it was born only a few days or weeks ago!"

"We are standing up now so that pregnant person can sit down and rest their body."

"Your preschool class had baby bunnies this year—they grew inside their mommy's uterus, too!"

"Only grown-ups have babies grow in their bodies—kids don't, because their bodies aren't ready yet."

The goal of this phase isn't so much to answer questions as it is to put the Foundations into practice—particularly Curiosity. It shows your child that you yourself are curious about the world and observing what happens around you, and reinforces that they are safe to talk to you about what they see in the world.

Phase Two: What Are Babies Made Of? (ages 2 to 5)

Once kids are used to recognizing what a pregnant body looks like, the questions about the origins of That Baby in There start to come up. This is when you might get your first "where do babies come from?," but it's important to recognize that most kids aren't asking for the whole story at this point. Consent for knowledge and verifying what question you're answering is vital here. I recommend starting *all* body talk conversations at this phase, regardless of the age of the child, particularly if it is the first time the child has expressed any interest in the topic.

"Where do babies come from?"

Young/early language child: "Babies are made when two cells combine and help each other grow into a baby! Cells are like your LEGOs, except cells build people!"

Slightly older/more verbal child: "It's a super cool process! When a baby is made, there are two cells that each have only a part of the instructions to make a baby. So, the cells combine together, and they share their information and work together to make a baby!"

In my experience, young children are satisfied with this level of answer and will not ask you to elaborate until they are ready for more information. Sometimes, however, children express a desire to know more in that moment, at which point you can move to the next phase by asking what more they would like to know.

Phase Three: How Does the Baby Come Out? (ages 3 to 6)

Generally speaking, when referring to where pregnancies occur, most children and adults use more colloquial language: "in her belly" or "in her tummy," to name two of the most common descriptors. Because of this tendency to blur the lines about what is happening and where it's happening, children can draw some pretty interesting conclusions about both how a baby got *into* where it is, and how that baby gets *out*.

"*(horrified stare)* Did she EAT the baby?!"

"I'm pretty sure my mom is going to poop out the baby soon *(confident nod)*."

As adults we know that neither of those assertions is true, but for children, these conclusions are the *peak* of logic. They are utilizing what those in psychology refer to as schema, or systems of organization that help them make sense of their world by fitting new information into a structure similar to what they already understand. And if they've been told that babies grow "in a tummy," the same place that connects their mouths and their bowels, it makes sense:

- A baby grows in a belly.
- Things go into the belly through the mouth.
- Things leave the belly through the butt.
- Therefore, a baby has to be eaten to end up in the belly and must be pooped out to be born.

In order to help children build new schema that are both more accurate and helpful in understanding future concepts (as well as their own body), it is vital that we help kids understand that babies grow in a uterus—a special organ made of muscle that protects the baby—and that babies come out via one of two ways: a vaginal birth or a C-section.

How Do Babies Come Out?

Young/Early Language Child

Parents, especially parents expecting the arrival of a sibling for their young child, are likely to be asked questions repeatedly for weeks: "How is the baby coming out?" "How will it get out?" "How will it get here?" It can be helpful for both your child and your frustration levels to have a simple, accurate answer that can be supplied automatically, like "Sometimes they are pushed out, sometimes they need help." This both answers the question and offers some comfort for a child who is noticing how much everything around them is changing. Sometimes a question isn't really a request for information, but a way of seeking reassurance that their caregiver knows what will happen, and that what will happen isn't something to worry about.

For children who *are* seeking information, or who want a more thorough answer, the following is an accurate and age-appropriate answer to the question:

"Babies are born! They can come out of the pregnant person's vagina, which is a part of their body in between their legs, or they can come out from a surgery."

Slightly Older/More Verbal Child

> "The process of a baby being born is called giving birth. Remember how we talked about how people with a uterus also have a vagina and a vulva? Well, when people with a uterus give birth, the strong muscles of the uterus help push the baby down through the vagina and out of the body! Some babies are also born in a different way called a C-section. A C-section is where a doctor very carefully cuts into the uterus and helps the baby come out through the cut they made, which gets closed up after the baby is out!"

Phase Four: Where Do the Cells Come From? (ages 4 to 6)

As kids move into a more concrete and increasingly complex understanding of the world, they start to recognize when their deck is missing cards, so to speak. They start to catch on when answers are simplified for them, and they seek to increase their knowledge of the nuance of the situations they're discussing. Because of this, one of the pieces of the "where do babies come from?" puzzle is helping kids understand what kinds of cells are combining in a uterus, and where those cells come from. This is not likely a conversation you'll have to have with a very young child—instead, children ask these questions as they get older, and they may come rapid-fire as part of other conversations.

Cells from the Parents

> "There are only two kinds of cells that can make a baby—one is called a sperm, and one is called an egg. The sperm comes

from someone with a penis—like your (dad/papa/parent/etc.). The egg comes from someone with a uterus—like your (mom/mama/parent/etc.). Since we knew we needed one of each kind, we agreed that we would share our cells to make you."

Cells from Donors

"There are only two kinds of cells that can make a baby—one is called a sperm, and one is called an egg. The sperm comes from someone with a penis. The egg comes from someone with a uterus. To make a baby, there has to be one of each, so in order to make you [insert circumstance here—one donor cell into parent or surrogate, two donor cells into parent or surrogate, etc.]."

The follow-up questions during this phase may center around the attributes of the cell:

An EGG?! Like a chicken?

No, not a chicken egg, a people egg! It is so tiny you can't see it with your eyes, and it doesn't have a hard shell like a chicken egg, either.

What does an egg look like?

Kind of like it sounds—round, like a chicken egg! But it's SUPER tiny—you can't see it with your eye, you have to use a microscope!

What does a sperm look like?

Sperm are similar to eggs in that they're roundish, but they have a little tail that helps them swim to where they need to be. They are *also* super tiny—even tinier than an egg!

Why do you need one of each?

Because sperm and eggs only have part of the information to make a person, not all of it! Imagine trying to build [LEGO set/furniture/train set] with only half of the instructions and half of the pieces—would it work? Probably not! The two kinds of cells have to combine to make sure they have all the instructions and all the pieces needed to make a baby!

Early to Middle Childhood Scripts

Phase Five: How Do the Cells Get Into the Uterus? (ages 5 to 7)

This is the part of the discussion that everyone seems to dread, and that I am not even allowed to put on social media for fear of it being taken down. Which is a real shame, because as we've established, it's incredibly valuable to normalize talking with our children about our bodies and how they work.

In this phase of information sharing with children at this age, I believe it is *crucial* to lead with consent for knowledge. Let your child know that you are happy to answer their questions, but also that they may have follow-up questions or Big Feelings about the knowledge you are about to impart. If the child asserts that they do, indeed, feel ready to hear this information, consider starting by sharing the method used to create your child. Once you have shared the information, remind your child that you will continue to respect their boundaries around knowledge, *and* that they need to respect other people's boundaries, too. Part of being "old enough" to ask and have answers to questions that their friends may not have access to is knowing who they can share that information with.

Now you know how babies are made! Who can you talk about this with?

Uhhh . . . you?
Yes.

Dr. K?
Sure, if you have questions!

My other safe grown-ups?
Absolutely—they are your safe grown-ups in part because they know our family boundaries! [*You may consider verifying with your child who the safe grown-ups are, if this is a suggestion they make.*]

My friends?
Pump the brakes there, kiddo. Nope! This information is for their safe grown-ups to share with them, not you. If you are unsure if the person you want to talk to about this is okay, then you can always feel safe to ask me and I'll let you know!

Sex

Unlike in other parts of this book so far, in this section, I use very simplified, gendered language. Though the use of these words can (and should) be phased out as kids mature and develop a more advanced understanding of where babies come from, starting with this very basic language allows their understanding to scaffold over time. As children get older, you can swap out words like "mom" and "dad" for "person with a uterus" and "person with a penis" to help them develop nuance in their understanding of intersecting identities and different family structures. This inclusive language fosters a more complete understanding of the spectrum of people who exist in our world, and establishes a baseline of respect and understanding for our children as they grow.

> *First:* "Well, you know that there have to be two cells to make a baby, right? In order to make a baby, a mom and a dad have to decide to let their bodies touch when they're naked. Then the cell goes from the penis into the uterus and the baby grows!"
>
> *Second:* "When the grown-ups are trying to make a baby, the man and the woman use their swimsuit parts together to help the cell go from the penis into the uterus."
>
> *Third:* "Sex is when a man puts his penis into a woman's vagina so that a sperm cell can go into the uterus and combine with a cell called an egg, and once those cells are together, a baby can grow."

This conversation, in particular, often leads to a myriad of follow-up questions, some of which may be *very* unexpected:

Do people do that in the night, or in the day?
Whatever makes the two grown-ups feel comfortable!

Is that something people do at home? Or in their cars?
Usually this is something that happens at home.

Can only grown-ups do this?
Yup—only grown-ups should be having sex.

Do my FRIENDS know about this?!

They might, but remember—if your friends want to know, they should ask their caregivers.

Can I watch?

Nope! Sex is something grown-ups do in private—a kid should never be watching a grown-up have sex.

But . . . I think I saw people doing that [on the computer/in a movie].

You might have. Those kinds of [videos/movies] are for grown-up brains—your brain is safest learning about sex from other places like talking to me and exploring your own body for a while first.

Wait, THAT'S what you and Mom were doing?!

Well, yes. Like we talked about, though, that was a time when we wanted privacy. You didn't know that when you opened our door, and that's why you didn't get in trouble. But now you know, so you know that if our door is shut, you should always knock first!" [*This answer can hopefully circumvent the guilt pathway of "I should have known better!" because how could they have known?!*]

Do people have a baby every time they have sex?

No, there are lots of things that have to happen in the body for a baby to be made. But for lots of healthy adults, any time they have sex, they *might* be able to make a baby. [*This answer is both factual and begins to normalize the necessity of protection and prevention during sexual encounters.*]

But if they aren't having a baby, why are they having sex?
Because for most grown-ups, sex feels good for their bodies, and gives them happy feelings, too.

Intrauterine Insemination (IUI)

> *Medically Assisted:* "When we decided to have you, we went to a doctor to ask for help. The doctor helped us know when the eggs in [Mom's/our surrogate's] uterus might be ready, and then helped us use a special tool to put the sperm cells from [Dad/our sperm donor] into the uterus so that they could combine to make you!"

> *At-Home/Unassisted:* "When we decided to have you, we kept track of important information that helped us know when the eggs in [Mom's/our surrogate's] uterus might be ready, and then we used a special tool to put the sperm cells from [Dad/our sperm donor] into the uterus so that they could combine to make you!"

In Vitro Fertilization (IVF)

> "When we decided we wanted to have you, we asked for help from a doctor whose whole job is helping to make babies in a lab. We took some sperm cells from [dad/our sperm donor] and some eggs from [Mom/our egg donor] and the doctor combined them in a special container called a petri dish! Then after the doctor was sure that the cells were combined, they were moved from the petri dish into the uterus where you grew and grew until you were born!"

IUI and IVF follow-up questions are also common, and may include things like:

Where did the cells come from?

Each answer to this question is unique, just like each of you!

But wait, if the cell didn't come from you, are you really my [mom/dad/parent]?

Yes! I am very grateful to the person who shared their cell with us and helped you be made. And I am very happy that I get to help you become you with what I teach you and how I love you every day.

What If They Never Ask? (adolescence, or ages 8+)

So what do you do if your child just . . . never asks where babies come from? How do you approach the conversation with a child who blanches and bolts when you even tiptoe near the topics of romance or intimacy, or the dreaded idea of "doing it"? How do you handle it if your child is very clearly old enough to know but has so far evaded the conversation? Here are some ways you can start the conversation in a few different circumstances.

If a sense of curiosity or tendency to ask questions has not been established

> **AGES 8+:** You still have time to normalize curiosity. Consider starting by pointing out where other kinds of babies come from. You could even frame it as a question: "So chickens lay eggs, and kangaroos have pouches, but cats have live babies. I wonder how they are all

different." By making it clear that the topic of reproduction in general isn't taboo, you may begin modeling to your child that they can ask you questions.

AGES 10+: Children at this age *need* to have at least basic information about how babies are made. If they haven't asked yet, then you as the parent should bring it up: "We've never really talked about where babies come from, and you will probably be learning about it in school soon. Are you comfortable talking with me about it?" If they say yes, then the conversation can proceed as illustrated earlier in the chapter (see page 146). If the child says no, then it's worth going to the final conversation in this section on page 160.

If your child has previously asked where babies come from and been told "I'll tell you when you're older"

If *you* postponed the conversation at some earlier point and your child hasn't brought it up again, I hate to break it to you, but it's on *you* to get the ball rolling: "Hey, remember when you asked me where babies come from and I said I'd tell you when you were older? Well, you're older now, so it's probably a good time for us to talk about it. Are you feeling ready?"

If your child thinks they already know where babies come from

Some kids have just extrapolated some idea based on what they might know about sea turtles or sharks (a psychological concept called magical thinking), some kids might've read something they weren't supposed to, and others really do already know. My favorite strategy is to flip the script. Become the student—let them teach you. What this will help you understand is what their perceived knowledge is, where they got the information, and how you can correct their understanding going forward. Ask your child to explain to you what they know and then have a conversation about what they got right, what they got wrong, and everything in between. This will not only strengthen their knowledge, it will also help you solidify that you are an accessible and safe point of contact for information seeking.

If your child has misinformation from you that you need to correct

In the course of developing this book, I received messages and comments from folks lamenting how they'd "screwed it up." How they panicked in the moment and leaned into a lie. How they wish they'd had a resource to guide them through the conversations. Maybe that's why you picked up this book—you're trying to course correct. Because—let's face it—sometimes the easiest answer is simply to lie to our children. I didn't say it was the *right* answer, but for some of us, it's the easiest one. The problem with lying to our kids is that we then have to correct the lie or risk having someone else correct it and losing our children's trust as a result. If your child is no longer wondering where babies came from because you've provided misinformation, it is your responsibility to correct that misinformation. This will come with a healthy dose of self-effacement: "Hey, I wanted to let you know that when you asked me where babies come from and I said that they were delivered by the stork, that wasn't true. I didn't want to tell you because I didn't know that you were ready, but I know now that you're responsible enough. And I trust you with this information. I know your brain can handle it, and I know you won't share it with people who aren't ready for it."

I will just add here that because your child is an autonomous human, there is no way to guarantee that they will not share the information with other kids. I have found that checking in with children and reinforcing who can and should share that information is more helpful than frequently reminding them that they shouldn't be sharing it.

If your child doesn't want the information

As I've said in previous portions of this book, sometimes your kids don't want the information from *you*. It's not because they don't trust you or because there is something wrong with your bond; some kids are just very private human beings. They feel uncomfortable acknowledging their own existence, much less their own sexuality. If you have one of these kids, be incredibly careful and pick your battles about what needs to be discussed. If it's a biological concept and an answer is available in book form, hand them the book. If they might feel more comfortable getting this information from a trusted adult like a doctor, allow the doctor to explain it. Choose which topics require a discussion with you, and for the others, allow them the out of getting the information from a different source that you trust to be accurate, safe, and responsible. Respecting your child's autonomy and privacy will go so much further than forcing them to feel they have to hide from you lest they be driven into uncomfortable conversations.

CHAPTER 8: IN BRIEF

One of the most universal experiences in parenting is being faced with the question "where do babies come from?" and having to decide the best way to answer it. Like with most other topics related to bodies, reproduction can and should be presented to children factually with age-appropriate information that can be scaffolded and reinforced as they grow.

Key Takeaways

- Babies grow in a uterus, which is a special organ made of muscle whose job is to grow babies.

- Babies are made with two cells—a sperm and an egg. These cells combine their information and grow into a baby.

- Babies come out either through a person's vagina or through an incision in their stomach called a C-section.

- The cells required to make a baby come from one person with a penis and one person with a vagina, and can be combined inside someone's body through sex or through intrauterine insemination, or outside someone's body through in vitro fertilization.

- For younger children: Only grown-ups should be having sex.

- Sex does not always result in a baby—sex can also happen because it feels good—but people should remember that most vaginal sex *can* result in a baby, so they should plan accordingly and use protection if they do not want to have a baby.

PART 3

SPECIFICS

O nce you get the hang of the Mechanics conversations, it kind of feels like the world is your oyster. You feel confident using biological terms, you know how to keep things positive—your kid knows they can ask you anything, they're curious, and they have the power to consent to knowledge. For a while it feels like everything is coming up roses . . . and then the Specifics show up.

The Specifics are conversations that need to be had when kids start *really thinking* about the fact that sex requires at least two people. Because if there are two people, and one of those people is them, then . . . the questions start popping up like weeds The following chapters are designed to help you start conversations about how the Mechanics work in the context of interpersonal relationships—how people get from exploring *themselves* to exploring *each other.*

Just as they were in the Mechanics chapters, the Foundations are going to be instrumental in navigating these conversations. Keeping unconditional positive regard at the forefront of every discussion is going to help ease a child's mind as they begin trying to grapple with what exactly it means to be a person who can be in a relationship. Curiosity will allow a child to ask the questions that come into their mind, even if they do so through the lens of a hypothetical "friend" rather than admitting they are the ones wondering. Curiosity, too, can help a parent encourage a child to consider the morals that come up outside the context of simple Mechanics: "What might you do if your friend is drunk at a party and you see them walking into a bedroom with someone else?"

Consent for knowledge becomes somehow both more nuanced and easier as children move into the Specifics conversations. It is more nuanced because children in middle childhood need to know different levels of information than children in later adolescence. But it's simpler because as children reach the age where Specifics become more interesting to them, they will sometimes just . . . ask you the question, and you can answer it.

As you embark on these discussions, please do not hesitate to continue reviewing the Mechanics chapters. As your kids develop a broader understanding of interpersonal relationships, they may want to revisit some of the simpler information and apply their new understanding to how things work. Remember your boundaries and enjoy the adventure!

CHAPTER 9

The Feels

My parents met in the fall of 1969. My dad, a twenty-one-year-old army veteran newly home from Vietnam, had spent a large part of his first months home trying to recover from what he had witnessed during his time overseas. My mother, on the other hand, was a fresh high school graduate excited to branch out into life as an adult. The freshman mixer was *the* place to be on their college campus, so naturally both of them were there. My mom had just walked into the venue with her roommate and was surveying the room when she spotted him. He was six feet six and lean from his army service, with dark hair and a thick moustache. She turned to her roommate and pointed him out: "See that man over there? That's the man I'm going to marry." She did what any savvy woman would do: She loosened the belt that was delicately balanced on her hips accessorizing her sheath dress—and sauntered across his path. She timed her steps just right, and bam—the belt slipped over her hips, down her legs, and landed on the floor as she walked away. My dad didn't even know what hit him—he picked up the belt to hand it back to her, and the rest was history. They were engaged three months later and married a year after that.

They went on to have five kids, live in three states, and earn graduate degrees. My mom never hesitated to share the story of how they met, and my dad was forever leaving my mom little notes about how much he loved her and his family. There was a lot of love in the house where I grew up, and my parents were both really intentional about how they expressed that to their children—they both said they were going to be "huggin' and kissin'" parents. They wanted us to always feel comfortable coming to them for snuggles, climbing into their laps, or just generally seeking them out for physical comfort because neither of them had had that in abundance growing up.

My parents also made sure we understood that if we decided to share our lives with a partner, we should be aiming for a healthy, happy relationship like theirs. They never fought in front of us, they expressed their emotions effectively, and overall they modeled what a marriage could be when both people worked at it.

They were pretty ahead of their time, especially given where I grew up. As I've mentioned, they didn't shy away from the topic of sex—if we asked a question, they answered, and they were honest about sex being for making babies. I ask my friends now how much their parents taught them about sex and relationships, and for many, the answer was "Don't get knocked up or knock anyone up!" So I am grateful for how much information I got, and for the healthy modeling of an adult relationship. The problem was this: Sex was *almost exclusively* discussed in the context of a happy, loving, monogamous coupling. I don't remember it ever being explicitly stated, but I do remember internalizing that sex *could* happen outside of marriage, but it was *best* within it. So much better, in fact, that we shouldn't ever discuss *why* it was better—just take it as fact.

To be clear, I do not fault my mother for not tackling the intimacy discussion—it certainly was not something she had modeled for her, and the conversations she had with my siblings and me about sex were instrumental in keeping us as safe and happy as we were. But by not talking about intimacy, particularly sexual intimacy, her teachings missed a key part of what makes a happy, healthy partnership.

Yes, it feels weird to consider talking about intimacy with my children. But when you step back and think about it for a second, books, television, and movies are already giving them the information . . . only less accurately and significantly less helpfully! The examples of relationships that our kids are getting from the media they consume can be not only inaccurate, but harmful, too. In one of my psychopathology classes, a student shared a clip from a show called *Miraculous: Tales of Ladybug & Cat Noir*. In the clip, one of the characters was shown dealing with her attraction to someone by memorizing his schedule, stealing his cell phone, and manufacturing ways to bump into him in public. It was *appalling* that no one on the show called the behavior what it was: stalking. I went home that night and made sure I had a conversation with my children about what love and relationships look like, because heaven forbid they ever see something like that show and think stalking = love.

By making the definitions of both intimacy and relationships very clear, it becomes much easier for our kids to develop a gauge for what healthy relationships look like for *them*. Imagine how much more comfortable our kids would be if, rather than trying to guess and using the often questionable representations of young relationships in media, they had frequent and thoughtful conversations about their expectations and needs with the adults who care about them the most.

You might be struggling to talk to your kids about intimacy because we usually associate intimacy with romantic relationships, but intimacy is vital to humans all throughout their development. At its most basic, intimacy is the bond one individual forms with another (or others) in which they feel understood, respected, cared for, and comfortable sharing emotions and expressing private thoughts and feelings. None of those feelings are inherently romantic or sexual (and not everyone experiences romantic or sexual feelings, anyway)—they can be felt by people in relationships of many different kinds.

Though there is variation in the research, intimacy can generally be broken down into four different types: emotional, mental, spiritual, and physical. In all four types, individuals feel accepted and understood, and establish a willingness to communicate because of trust. However, each type of intimacy is formed through different domains. Emotional intimacy is closeness of feeling; sharing how you feel and hearing how somebody else feels; and feeling comfortable to express your emotions openly. Mental or intellectual intimacy is the sense that you can share your ideas and thoughts with another person; that you can explore big ideas together, or that the other person will help you grow by helping you think about things nonjudgmentally. Spiritual intimacy is closely related to both emotional and mental intimacy, but is tied specifically to a feeling that you can share your innermost beliefs—your purpose, your spiritual beliefs, or your religious beliefs—with another person without judgment. The other person may not have the same beliefs, but there is a sense that you are able to express those beliefs without fear of losing your connection. Finally, physical intimacy means feeling respected and safe while being physically close to someone. This includes what most people first think of when they hear the term "intimacy"—sex. But sex isn't the *only* form of physical intimacy, and sex isn't *always* an expression of physical intimacy.

Understanding the different types of intimacy and recognizing their influence on both platonic and romantic relationships is an important lesson for us, and for our children. In early and middle childhood, it helps children understand the purpose of friendship. We can ask "Why are the people who are in your life in your life?" Think about the friendships you've had throughout your life—the good ones and the bad ones. The good ones usually have one of the forms of intimacy established—they make us feel emotionally seen, intellectually stimulated, spiritually fulfilled, or physically safe. Do you have people in your life who provide none of these feelings of safety, security, or growth? If they are around you, taking up your time and energy without fulfilling any of those needs . . . should they be around? As our children navigate the often treacherous waters of adolescent friendships, having a solid grasp on the purpose of friendship can help them identify their true friends and separate themselves from the ones who are in their circle simply because of proximity. Taking it one step further, as they get old enough to consider picking romantic partners, they can ask themselves the same questions: *Does my romantic partner tick at least one intimacy box? Have I hit the jackpot and found someone who ticks all four boxes? And is that a two-way street—does my partner feel a sense of intimacy with me?*

As our children spread their wings and begin dating, it's important that they realize a long-term partnership requires all four levels of intimacy, not just physical intimacy, even though their biology is driving their hormones toward that physical fulfillment. Conveying to our children that the *other* forms of intimacy contribute significantly to a healthy relationship can help them make more fulfilling choices. They may even choose to delay sexual encounters to determine if their chosen partner provides other forms of intimacy before moving on to explore sexual intimacy.

In addition to intimacy, some theorists study the concept of love and its various forms within relationships. Psychologist and psychometrician Robert Sternberg proposed what he called the triangular theory of love, which states that the forms of love are based in three domains: intimacy (a sense of a closeness), passion (physical attraction and related phenomena like sex), and decision/commitment to the relationship (a decision that love exists between the people, and if the relationship lasts, a commitment to maintain it). These factors can exist on their own or combine to form seven different forms of love, and all forms of love can grow into each other and change over time:

> Intimacy alone without passion or commitment is known as liking
> or friendship.
> Passion without intimacy or commitment is called infatuation.
> Commitment without passion or intimacy is called empty love.
> Passion and intimacy with no commitment is called romantic love.
> Intimacy and commitment with no passion is called companionate love.
> Passion and commitment with no intimacy is known as fatuous love.
> Love that includes passion, intimacy, and commitment—the most "complete"
> and often idealized form of love—is called consummate love.

Thankfully, intimacy, love, and relationships are like most other sensitive and complex topics—they can be discussed in small bites over time. There's no need to navigate one big sit-down talk that covers everything, mostly because that would be both ineffective and impossible! No, frequent check-ins about the following topics, along with modeling your *own* priorities, values, and healthy relationships (both platonic and romantic) will help show your child what they should be aiming for as they navigate intimacy.

Sample Scripts

To Thine Own Self Be True (all childhood)

Checking in with our children and helping them understand who they are—what their core values and beliefs are—is difficult to do when we haven't figured out what our *own* core values and beliefs are. All too often I see parents who are distraught over a choice their child has made—quitting a sport, joining an activity, ending a friendship—without reflecting on why *they* are attached to their child's choice.

When my eldest child tried—and was indifferent toward—basketball, I was sad. I knew he was bound to be pretty tall—over six feet—and basketball has a long legacy in my family. I tried for a bit to ignite the passion for basketball in him—we played at open gym, would shoot around outside when we got the chance, and talked about the fundamentals of the game. He engaged in all those activities with gusto, and he was pretty good, too! But when I signed him up for a basketball camp or asked if he wanted to join the rec team, the most enthusiasm I got was an indifferent shrug. He would do it if I made him, but he certainly wasn't excited about it. When I finally gave in and asked what made him like basketball but not want to *do* basketball, he said, "The people. The other boys on the team aren't very kind and make me feel bad when I make mistakes. I don't want to be with them."

Well, crud. Now I was at a crossroads. I didn't want him to internalize that you should quit what you enjoy just because other people suck, but I also didn't want him to learn that Mom was going to force him to be around people he didn't like just because he kind of liked basketball (and Mom *really* liked basketball). We had a heart-to-heart, and as we talked, I had to keep this one question central in my mind: *What is right for* him? He talked to me about what he liked: He liked dribbling with Mom. He liked shooting with Mom. He liked open gym . . . with Mom. When it came to activities he enjoyed *without* Mom, he said he loved swimming, theater, and playing D&D with his friends. He had a clear head on what *he* valued, and I needed to honor that he could make decisions for himself about his free time. I needed to realize that my attachment to basketball was rooted in my *own* passion for the sport, and in some fantasy I had about cheering for him in a "traditional" sport. I hadn't recognized that I could cheer for him in countless other arenas that would make him so much happier than basketball ever could. I was a little bit sad that I might not have anyone to cheer for from the bleachers in a packed gymnasium, but I was significantly more proud that I had a child who was not only aware of what he wanted, but willing to advocate for himself to the most powerful adult he knew at the time—his mom.

As he's grown, we've continued touching base about how his core values intersect with his physical and developmental needs. He hasn't been allowed to ditch *all* sports, even though he doesn't love to compete, because it's good for his development to remain physically active and learn how to operate in a team environment. But rather than a sport like basketball, he has chosen the swim team as his "I'm going to learn about being a high school athlete" home. And as the results of his other decisions—both good and bad—play out, he can use the discussions we've had about his values and needs as an ever-evolving manual to help him become the adult he wants to be.

Checking in and making these conversations intentional has also helped me understand him so much better than I would have otherwise. I know the answers to questions like "What makes you happy?" I could list what he would say if I asked him "How do you like to spend your time?" He is prepped and ready to answer when I ask "What makes you feel appreciated? What makes you feel safe? When do you feel the best? What makes you sad? What do you do when you're feeling scared?" Though there have been times when he has made choices in direct contrast to his core values—everyone makes mistakes—when the consequences of those choices came back around, ultimately, it was those values *and* his sense of safety in coming to me for help that navigated him back to the course he wanted for himself.

My hope for my children—and for all children—is that as they leave childhood and enter the adult world they have a sense of what matters to them, *and* a willingness to pause and check in with themselves as they grow. Because those skills will be paramount in maintaining healthy, happy relationships with their friends, coworkers, family, partners, and, ultimately, their own children.

What Makes a Good Relationship? (ages 11+)

The world is full of people—gross, right? Just all these people with their own dreams and goals and wants and needs and agendas and flaws. I mean, it makes sense that *we* have all of those things, but when you zoom out and think about how there are literally eight billion other people on this planet who are just like that? It's almost too much to consider. Because that means that beyond knowing themselves, our children need interpersonal skills. They need to be able to not only assert their core values but understand and react to other people's core values. Thankfully, we can teach our kids these interpersonal skills, and also impress upon them how valuable these skills are in a partner.

Research on relationships is varied in type and scope, but most researchers, clinicians, and coaches agree on some fundamental building blocks of a healthy relationship. These blocks include communication, respect, trust, safety, honesty, responsibility, boundaries, and compatibility. As you read that list, you probably nodded to yourself and thought, *Heck yes, that's exactly my list*. Same! I agree—those are all essential concepts to have in a healthy relationship. Now . . . define them.

I'll wait.

This is where things get sticky. It might be easy enough to define safety—your partner doesn't hurt you. But safety also means that in addition to not hurting your *body*, they don't hurt you *emotionally, intellectually,* or *spiritually*. Your *all of you* has to be safe. Now we're edging from a definition into a conversation—of course. It's always a conversation with these dang kids.

Here are some examples of how you can start a conversation with your child about each of the aforementioned aspects of a healthy relationship. None of these scripts are exhaustive—as you know, these conversations are going to be ongoing—but they are a reasonable place to start.

Communication: "In a relationship, communication means that no one is expected to guess what the other person is thinking, feeling, or needing. The people in the relationship talk about what they expect—how much they will talk to each other, how much they will see each other, who will take care of shared responsibilities, and a lot of other things. Communication also means that if a mistake is made or someone doesn't hold up their end of the relationship, the people in the relationship will talk about it, not hold it in and let it bubble up later."

Respect: "A very basic definition of respect is that a person cares about the rights, feelings, desires, and core aspects of another person. You can also respect a person based on how they do their job or participate in activities. In a relationship, respect means that you care about another person's rights, feelings, desires, and core values *and* think about how your actions, thoughts, and values might impact them."

Trust: "When you trust someone, you know in your heart and in your mind that they care about you—that they will behave in a way that will not hurt you. You know that they will be reliable, tell you the truth, and be there for you within their own boundaries."

Safety: "A relationship needs to be safe, and that doesn't just mean that no one hurts each other's body. Obviously, I don't want you to be with someone who hits, pinches, slaps, punches, kicks, or does anything else that causes you physical harm. I *also* don't want you to be in a relationship with someone who hurts your mind—this is someone who makes you question if you're right all the time or makes you feel like you don't understand how the world works. They might make you think that you're always wrong or that people who *do* love you actually might *not* love you. You also need to have a relationship that is emotionally safe—you should not have to guess or wonder how your partner feels about you. You should be responsible for your actions and not be hurtful to your partner, *and* you should not be responsible for your partner's emotions or actions. And you need someone who is safe for you spiritually—someone who respects your spiritual beliefs and doesn't expect you to change in order to be with them."

Honesty: "We've talked a lot about what honesty means, right? How it means telling the truth when you're asked directly, but it also means making choices that are honest even if you're not going to be questioned about them. Remember when we went to the store and the clerk forgot to scan the soda under the cart? What did we do? We went back in and we paid for it—that's honesty, and it's also integrity. Honesty in a relationship means that the partners tell each other important things, silly things, interesting things, and even things that might be sad or might contribute to the other person having strong emotions, like bad news, or that one person might have changed how they feel about the other. Honesty isn't always easy, but it is almost always easier than dishonesty, especially in relationships."

Responsibility: "Responsibility in relationships is almost exactly like what responsibility is in our family—it's being willing to say 'I did that' or 'I didn't do that' or 'I should have done that.' It's knowing what you need to do to maintain the relationship, and being willing to ask if you *don't* know. It's also important to be responsible in other parts of your life, because if you are irresponsible in one part of your life, like work, it can make being responsible in your relationship harder."

Boundaries: "Boundaries in a relationship get portrayed incorrectly *a lot*. People sometimes think that boundaries are about what each person in the relationship can or can't do—'My girlfriend can't wear those kinds of clothes' or 'My boyfriend can't talk to other girls—but those are *not* boundaries. Those kinds of statements are controlling behavior, and they are *not* part of a healthy relationship. Instead, boundaries are about what an individual person is comfortable with and will accept in a relationship—for example, a boundary might be 'I am not comfortable with a partner who wants to hide that we are dating, so if you are unwilling to acknowledge that we are partners, I can't be with you right now.' The person is saying, 'This is what I can accept, and if it doesn't

happen, then *I* will make this change.' If the partner wants
to change their behavior, they can, but they do not have to.
People can have boundaries about lots of things, but many
healthy relationships have boundaries about how disagree-
ments get handled, personal space, identity, and expectations
or goals. For example, your dad and I agree that we will not
yell at each other even if we are really mad. This is because
neither of us will listen to people yelling at us. We made it a
rule in our relationship that we talk, not yell. And if we feel
like we cannot talk right then, we tell the other person so and
take a five-minute break."

Compatibility: "Most of the other parts of what make a
good relationship feel really serious, right? They feel like big
ideas that take practice and that people can screw up—and
you're right. They're all pretty in-depth, and yes, people do
screw them up, even when they have a lot of practice. You'll
get better as you get bigger. *But* the cool thing is that the last
feature of a healthy relationship is actually pretty easy—it's
compatibility! Compatibility is how people in relationships
get along. Do they have similar goals? Do they care about
what the other person likes? For me and your dad, one of
the things that made us really compatible was that we both
loved to laugh, but we also loved to talk about big ideas. We
used to read interesting articles and scientific literature and
spend lots of time talking about what we learned. We were

compatible *intellectually*. We also shared a similar approach to emotions and communication—how we talked to each other about our feelings worked well. We had our own identities— we both had interests that the other person didn't share—but since we both valued learning, we were able to hear about the thing we weren't necessarily invested in ourselves because we invested in learning."

What Do *You* Need from Your Relationship? (ages 11+)

So now that we've set up the expectations about what a healthy relationship looks like, it's time for our kiddos to reflect on what *they themselves* need, rather than what they think they're *supposed* to need. How many of us can think back on an early relationship where we were less than in tune with our own needs, and it ended up being at best unsatisfactory, or at worst harmful? From my own early dating experiences, I can remember being shamed for "calling too much," being told I was a "prude" for not wanting to try things sexually, and thinking that I needed to keep my "nerdy" thoughts to myself because they were boring or embarrassing. As I got older, I realized that most of those feelings came from the fact that I was not prioritizing or even really thinking about what *I* needed. The only "need" I had identified in the relationship was for it to exist—for someone to want me.

I encourage my children and the children I work with to think about communication, space, time, affection, commitment, and any other attributes of a relationship that they can identify: "How much do you think a happy couple talks to each other? How much time do you think a teenager should spend talking to their partner instead of doing other activities? How do you feel about holding hands in public? What about hugging? How about kissing? Would you stop being friends with Sam if your new partner said that they weren't comfortable with you being friends with them? How would you respond to that? We talk when you're mad—how do you think you and a partner should handle conflict?" I discussed earlier that children learn a lot from what is modeled to them, both in their lives and in media, and that particularly in the case of media, the modeling isn't spectacular. As a caregiver, you have the power to encourage your kids to challenge the narratives they've been shown. If kids can spend time reflecting on these ideas and discover where their personal values and morals turn into preferences and boundaries, they can spend time practicing how to communicate these boundaries to their future partners. As with everything, these conversations will evolve as your child grows—a twelve-year-old is unlikely to have the same attitude about public displays of affection as a seventeen-year-old. And as these conversations evolve, so will your child's understanding of their boundaries and ability to maintain them.

Hide Your Flaws Until After the Wedding! (ages 11+)

I'm sure several of you reading this book read the last passage and thought, *Oh jeez, I absolutely had crappy early relationships like that—I don't even recognize the person I was back then.* So many of us Gen X and millennial parents were fed narratives that included the Dramatic Metamorphosis: Some perfectly fine character would have a makeover—of their appearance, their personality, their self-expression—and *suddenly*, they were "hot" and "datable." They also made it seem like the primary goal of high school should be graduating . . . and getting laid. The messaging was clear: There is a right way to be attractive, and the result of that attractiveness is to get some. The truth is that most teens in the US wait until seventeen to have sex, and that only about half of teenagers have had sex during their high school years, which flies in the face of what media told us was the norm. Thankfully, many of us figured out as we got older that we did not need to change ourselves to be with someone. This was great, but we also figured out that we might never find our someone.

This can be really difficult for young people to stomach. We have biological drives toward partnership—we *want* to find someone to be with, even if it's not forever. For those of us who are ... unconventional ... in our presentation, whether that's being an incredibly tall woman or having an eclectic sense of style (or both ... hi, yes, I'm describing myself), it can be so hard to watch your more conventional peers partner up and at least get to *practice* being someone's love interest. This feeling of envy can become jealousy and resentment—people who feel like their singleness is involuntary and that they are somehow "owed" the attention of the people they are attracted to. (We definitely want to nip those feelings in the bud, because they are not healthy—no one owes you attention.) But the feeling of envy can swing another direction and become the feeling that if you just changed *these few things* about yourself, you'd be loveable. Just get skinnier. Just wear the right clothes. Just agree to have sex.

Danger zone. Pump the brakes, kiddo. It is *so hard* to become content with being single, I won't deny it. It took me a long time. Eventually, though, I came to understand the truth: that many of us may not find our people until we're older, especially if we're coming from somewhere with a limited pool of potential partners. But staying true to ourselves—our interests, our goals, and our values—is so much more satisfying than compromising and settling for someone who doesn't actually know us. And even if we never find our forever partner—if we don't happen to cross paths—being true to ourselves means we can surround ourselves with people who appreciate us for who we are. Friends who value us for our communication, respect, trust, safety, honesty, responsibility, and boundaries, and who are compatible with the *real* us.

How Do I Know If I Like Someone? (ages 11+)

Having this talk with a kid can feel a bit like trying to walk through a hall of mirrors wearing those anti-drunk-driving goggles—it's disorienting and complicated and you might end up smashing your face. The honest truth is that our kids' preferences grow and change along with our kids, so rather than helping them identify exactly what they're looking for in a person and saying "you will feel like *this* when you have a crush on someone," we should be letting them know that understanding their own attraction depends on knowing themselves. For some people, initial attraction is almost solely based on appearance: "That man is literally the hottest human being I've ever seen, I'm going to ask him out." Some folks do not feel initial attraction until they get to know someone: "It's so interesting, she got more and more attractive the more time we spent together." Some people never really find themselves attracted to anyone: "I like to hang out, but the idea of making out with any of them is just . . . It just seems like there are better things to do than mushing our faces together." As caregivers, we must allow our kids space to figure out how they make decisions about relationships, and support them as they make those decisions, even if those decisions lead to tears and the realization that they need to do something different next time.

"Dating when you're a young person is mostly about figuring out what you might want in a partner, and what you absolutely can't work with. So long as you are being true to yourself, respecting boundaries, and being safe, I think dating can be a great thing. You don't *have* to date—you can choose to focus on other things—but you can date if you want."

"Just . . . ignore all the shows that paint dating as some sort of fraught, melodramatic, super-serious thing when you're a teenager. It doesn't have to look like that—most of that drama is from people not communicating well at all. If you and the person you're dating are talking about boundaries and expectations, you won't avoid *all* conflict, but it's not going to look like an episode of *Euphoria*."

"Some media portrays high school relationships as really dramatic—all cheating and two-timing and dumping people in dramatic fashion. They do not have to be that way—it's not a necessary or expected part of having a relationship, it's literally just to make 'interesting' watching. Please remember when you are dating people that they are people, not characters in media, and that if they are leaning into more drama than you are comfortable with, you can set boundaries and protect your heart."

Playing Dress Up (ages 11+)

I have been over six feet tall (193 centimeters, to be exact) since I was eleven years old. I went from looking very much like a little girl to looking almost like an adult in the span of a summer. This has been true for many of the children in my family—they grow tall and physically mature very quickly, while their preteen brains try valiantly to keep up. This genetic trait is part of what has shaped my opinion on how I talk to my kids about clothing and appearance.

When kids are small, clothes are almost entirely practical—they are used for self-expression, yes, but they are mostly chosen by how functional they are for play. I don't do short shorts, because it's impossible to go down a slide effectively when your legs are sticking to it; I don't do tank tops or crop tops because they mean more surface area to which I have to apply sunscreen; I don't do dry-clean-only clothes because there's no way I'm taking stuff to the cleaners. But as my kids have gotten older and their opinions on clothes have gotten louder, I've had to reflect on what I will buy and allow my children to wear, and where I'll draw the line.

I wish that all children could wear whatever they wanted and not have any unsolicited attention paid to them. In my dream world, dating, relationships, and courting would be driven much more by verbal communication and much less by how we present ourselves. But that's not the world we live in—we live in a world where, good or bad, what we wear sends messages. I know that if I'm looking to bolster my self-esteem a bit, I can post a "thirst trap" online and be told I'm pretty. I know that if I want to avoid being hit on, I can wear sweats and a high bun when I go to the grocery store. I want to be *very clear* here—there is *no* style of dress that *ever* "asks for" or "encourages" sexual harassment or sexual assault. Period. But to say that we can't or don't manipulate our appearance to get more or less attention is disingenuous.

But that level of understanding—knowing that changing what I look like influences the attention I get from the outside world—wasn't something I understood fully when I started looking more like an adult. And that, again, was true for many of the kids in my family—they looked much more like a grown-up than they were, and they didn't fully understand the messages their appearance might be sending. If the same physical development timeline holds true for my kid, how should I, as their parent, navigate the way I dress them? How can I help them express themselves as they grow into their adult bodies, while still protecting their kid brains? Like most of the decisions I make in parenting, I look to developmental science, in addition to my own lived experience and personal values, to help shape my opinion. What I've landed on is this: My children will dress for the world we live in, not for the one I wish they did, and they will do so until they understand self-expression and attention. Though I wish I could change the world so my children could wear whatever they want and get no unwanted attention whatsoever, I recognize that's *not* the world we live in, and I know my children are not the cudgel that will bring about that change.

> "I love back to school shopping with you! You know my favorites are the office supplies, but clothes are so fun, too. Hey, we should pop over there and check out the bras and camisoles. You're getting to the age where those are going to become staples when you're out and about. You don't have to wear a bra if we can't find one that's comfy, but you do have to make sure you have something to support your growing body, like a camisole or tank top. We can go check out what feels best."

"Oofda, those pants are getting short on you! We're going to have to go pick out different ones this year now that you're growing so much. Let's check out a different style this time—those ones were comfy, but now that you're growing, we gotta make sure we pick something that doesn't bind up or chafe around your penis, and also something that lays reasonably when you're standing up. I bet we can find some pants that are comfy *and* cut just right if we look!"

"I know you love rainbows, and I'm glad you do. You also have both of your ears pierced, which is fantastic. Those choices in accessories are part of expressing who you are, and that's lovely. You might not know this, but now that you look more mature, those accessories might be interpreted as you being part of the queer community. You know I'm going to love you and support you always, so if you are a member of the community—cool. You never have to stop wearing the things you like but know that you might get some high fives or appreciative nods from people because your accessories tell them you're a safe human. And given that you don't exactly like to 'people,' that might be more human interaction than you're anticipating. Just thought you ought to know!"

Before You "Do It" (ages 13+)

Unfortunately, the same media that's painted teen relationships as mini Shakespearean tragedies has also perpetuated the idea that sex is both meaningless *and* the ultimate goal—I think about every teen movie made in the early and mid-2000s and feel so sad for the messages I got as a young person. As a parent, this is frustrating in part because it complicates already complex topics—the intersections of sexuality, romance, attraction, and personal readiness. Conversations about these topics are going to be highly influenced by factors exclusive to you—things like your values, spiritual beliefs, location, culture, and more. The following scripts express my own feelings toward the topics of intimacy, sex, relationships, and communication, and serve as a good jumping-off point for you to reflect how you might tailor these scripts for use with your own children.

> "There are lots of people who think that sex is the most intimate thing you can do with a partner. And for some people, that is true—they feel like sex is the ultimate culmination of a relationship. But it's important to me that you understand that there are several steps for partners to go through *before* they have sex, and that those steps are *also* very intimate. Getting to know someone's likes, dislikes, fears, dreams, and private thoughts is a form of intimacy that is not physical. There is also physical intimacy that doesn't involve sex, like being willing to get undressed in front of a person who knows a lot about your private thoughts. There is also touching another person's body in ways that they like or that make them feel aroused—including touching their external genitals. All of those are ways to be intimate with a partner that do not include penetrative or oral sex."

If You Can't Talk About It . . . (ages 13+)

One of the best and most powerful self-reflective tools I was ever given for maintaining my own physical and emotional health has a mystical origin. The phrase was "If you can't talk to your partner about it, should you be doing it?" I called my sister to ask where it came from, because I remember hearing the message from at least a couple of my safe grown-ups when I was a kid. She couldn't remember who said it first, either (it might have been her, if I'm honest), but we both held on to it like a flashlight in the dark. It was simple and straightforward—if you didn't feel comfortable talking to your partner about your boundaries and needs in sexual situations, perhaps you should reflect on if you were actually comfortable enough to be having sex with them. Not only did this mantra help steer me out of situations when I realized I felt less than prepared to sleep with someone, it also helped me confirm when I *was* ready—because I felt like I could voice what I needed to my partner, and therefore did.

> "One of the best ways to determine if you're ready to have sex with your partner is to see if you feel comfortable talking about *all* aspects of sex with them. Do you know your body enough to know what you like? Do you feel comfortable telling your partner what you like? If they ask you to try something you don't think you'll like, do you feel comfortable enough to say no? All of these are good questions to ask yourself before you decide if you want to have sex with that person."

CHAPTER 9: IN BRIEF

As children grow, their relationships move from being highly based on proximity (relationships built with people they are close to physically) to being based on factors like communication, trust, respect, safety, honesty, responsibility, boundaries, and compatibility. Parents should talk to their children about how healthy relationships feature the aforementioned factors, as well as intimacy and love. Children should be encouraged to reflect on which attitudes, values, and behaviors in their friends and (later) their partners contribute to feelings of intimacy, commitment, and (someday) passion.

Key Takeaways

- Before embarking on romantic relationships or highly intimate friendships, it is valuable to identify what your child views as their core values and beliefs, as well as what makes them happy and fulfilled—help them develop and foster a sense of self.

- Intimacy is a sense of closeness and safety—whether spiritual, emotional, mental, or physical—with another person.

- Intimacy is integral to human experience, but is not necessarily easy to talk about with children.

- The triangular theory of love states that there are three key domains to love—intimacy, passion, and commitment—and that the levels of each domain in a relationship can change over time.

- Children should be encouraged to reflect on their relationships—both platonic and romantic—to determine how they are being impacted by the levels of intimacy and types of love.

- Social connectedness is valuable for maintaining resilience, so children should be encouraged to build relationships.

CHAPTER 10

Consent NOW

I t's dark, there's entirely too many people here, and I am not sure how we got to the point where he isn't wearing any pants. Not exactly a thought Kelsey had ever anticipated she would have running through her head, but there she was—about to be seventeen years old, in the apartment of a newish friend, with a boy she'd recently met whom she'd been "dating" for a few weeks.

That time of her life had been difficult—her mom had moved out almost two years before, her dad was recovering from being very ill, and she had spent the previous school year bouncing around to different houses with caregivers who were trying their best to keep the wheels turning in her life. Add the fact that she had been bullied extensively for not fitting traditional beauty standards, and you had a recipe for precarious relationships and ill-advised choices. Plus, she was a teenager—she was hardwired to make mistakes.

The newish friend had been helping Kelsey meet people and feel accepted during the summer of chaos. She couldn't tell me where they had met; they had gone to the same school, but the friend was a few years older—old enough, in fact, that she had her own apartment and much older friends. All Kelsey distinctly remembered was that one of her friend's friends brought a boy around who was maybe the most attractive boy she'd ever seen in real life: "He *legitimately* looked like a movie star." I feel for Kelsey like I feel for myself—sad for those younger versions of us, so desperate for romantic attention that it didn't matter if it was positive or negative.

Kelsey and the boy spent minimal time getting to know each other—he wasn't terribly talkative in the first place, they didn't spend tons of time alone, and they had almost nothing in common. But that didn't matter much to Kelsey at the time. The thing she was most interested in was that he wasn't embarrassed to be seen with her. At least not in front of the small group of people they spent time with. That he was interested in her *at all* was the only threshold she felt needed to be met.

As we look back on it now, she can see all the red flags: The perceived pressure (from him and others around her) to be together. The lack of communication but the feeling that she *had* to agree to physical closeness. "Not that he ever explicitly pressured or coerced me—the sense of duty was being supplied by the voice in my head," she said. There was very much a feeling of *He's going to dump me if I don't* . . . Which was how she ended up in the position she was telling me about—feeling like she was at a crossroads.

I had been in a very similar situation at about the same age, and I'm grateful that my story had a happy ending—the interaction stopped before anything regrettable happened, in part because of discussions I'd had with at least one caring adult in the year leading up to that summer.

Like many women my age, I was not immune to believing my worth was tied to how desirable I was in a relationship. An extension of that feeling was thinking that I would be more desirable the more passive or submissive or willing to make my partner happy I was. I know now how lucky I was to have the adults in my life that I did—I had been told for my entire childhood that I was a valuable and cherished person, no strings attached. I also understood that my autonomy was absolute—that my consent was *required* for a sexual encounter. But it wasn't until I had a conversation with my older sister that I fully understood: In order to consent, I had to be at least a *little bit* excited to do whatever I was consenting to.

For children raised with "no means no," we assume that the concept of consent should be fairly automatic. We assume they understand that bodily autonomy is nonnegotiable and that any physical encounter must include consent. What can become complicated is helping kids understand how their bodily autonomy interacts with other people's. That's where the FRIES framework (see page 57) comes into play. FRIES establishes that consent is freely given, reversible, informed, enthusiastic, and specific, sure, but what does that *mean* in real-world situations?

Teens most frequently have difficulty with the "freely given" and "reversible" aspects of the FRIES framework. We know that consent cannot be given if one party is impaired—if they are under the influence of drugs or alcohol—or if one party is a vulnerable human. But additionally, if there is a power imbalance or one party had to be convinced, coerced, or blackmailed into having sex, the agreement to engage in sex is not considered consent because the "yes" was not freely given. Emotional manipulation like "Don't you want to make me happy?" and "I just wish we loved each other as much as I thought we did" is something I've seen in far too many teen relationships, both in media and in my own life.

Similarly, many teens I've spoken with struggle to remember that consent is reversible. As I remind them, "Just because you've said yes previously, or you said yes even five seconds ago, doesn't mean that the 'yes' is permanent." I've heard teenagers say that in order to ensure that they are able to prove each person consented—to "provide receipts"—they will take photos or exchange text messages or sign a note that says they both agreed to sex. However, within the FRIES framework, we know that using text messages or phone calls as evidence that someone said yes to something is not the proof people think it is. Just because someone consented in a text message doesn't mean they consented in the moment, because they can reverse their consent at any point. Instead of thinking of a "gotcha" framework like tangible proof of consent, teens should be asked to reflect on why they might feel like they *need* tangible proof: "If you are concerned that you may need to prove your partner consented, are you sure that having sex with them is a good idea?"

This goes hand in hand with the "enthusiastic" message in the FRIES construct. When we discuss consent, lots of parents and caregivers focus on the "no" side of things—how to say no, what "no" means, what to do if you feel like someone isn't respecting your "no" and all of the things that can go wrong. These are all important conversations to have, particularly as we try to raise a generation of children who do not hurt each other by violating consent. But what some folks miss is that consent is inherently about "yes"—what you *do* want to partake in matters just as much as, if not more than, what you don't. And when we miss that discussion, we can end up with kids who feel like "yes" is wrong, or shameful, or should be avoided, and who also don't know that "yes" should be enthusiastic and engaged. Kids (like most people) aren't always great at seeing the areas in between the ends of the spectrum—it's either "all the way" or "absolutely not." So when an in-between thing happens, they might feel torn about whether it was a *good* thing. Highlighting for our kids that *they* are in control of their bodies and that they're allowed to say "yes" when they're ready is empowering, just as reminding them they can say "no" helps them feel safe. If we highlight their ability to provide (and accept) an enthusiastic "yes," they will hopefully recognize that proof of consent isn't necessary when consent is freely given, informed, enthusiastic, and specific.

I want to acknowledge right now that this might feel overwhelming. You might be reading all this and thinking you want to tell your kids "Just don't do it until you're adult and know better." I completely understand that desire, but remember that for most people, the drive for sexual contact is hardwired; humans are designed to want to keep going. It is evolutionarily beneficial for humans to want to make babies. And how do you make babies? With sexual contact. Add the fact that sexual contact feels good, and you have a recipe for people to get carried further into an interaction than they'd planned. There is an extra layer of risk for teens, whose brains aren't even done cooking and whose impulse control can be questionable at best. Having these (admittedly difficult) conversations is the best thing we can do to protect our children from their own biology. By helping our kids define where their boundaries and limits are and teaching them how to respect other people's boundaries, we give them the tools they need to find and be safe partners. As a caregiver and safe adult, you need to help your children know how to say yes and how to say no.

Sample Scripts

How Do You Know You're Ready (for Dating, Sex, and Otherwise)?

As we discussed earlier in the book, kids go through several stages of cognitive development. They also transition through periods of physical development, including puberty. Around age twelve, many children start to experience puberty and its associated hormones. These hormones are responsible for a myriad of changes, and also for a potential increase in sexual curiosity and the beginnings of sexual attraction. At around the same time, Piaget proposes that children begin to move into the formal operational stage of development where they can engage with higher-level thinking and logic. Because of these two changes—an increase in physical attraction and the ability to engage with more complex thoughts about boundaries, morals, needs, consequences, and behaviors—I arrived at what I call the Number Twelve Rule.

This rule states that, beginning at age twelve, children can begin to "date." This does not mean solo trips to Bali and their own hotel rooms. In the beginning, it means group outings with chaperones nearby in public places; it means finding out that your child is kissing and/or holding hands without freaking out; it means frankly discussing how to navigate sexual urges, peer pressure, and societal expectations with the knowledge that these are forces that may soon be impacting your child. Eventually, when a child has demonstrated that they understand how to advocate for themselves, how to have effective communication with you and with their partner, and how to accurately assess risk, consequences, and reward, they can move into more traditional dating (in my experience closer to ages fourteen, fifteen, and sixteen).

Are You Ready? (ages 11 to 13)

"We've talked a bit about dating and having crushes and stuff, and we have talked about how sex works. But we haven't really talked about how people decide when they're ready to date—to have a partner, kiss, hold hands, you know, all of that relationship stuff—or when they're ready to have sex. We have rules about when you are allowed to date—the number twelve rule that we've talked about—so you know that after twelve, you can start thinking about if you're ready to date. But did you know that some people will set goals about when they want to have sex? Some people say they want to wait until they're married, others want to be engaged first, and some people say they want to wait until they are a certain age. Right now, you are just starting puberty—your brain is changing a lot, and so is your body—so you are *not* ready to have sex. That will change as you get older, but for now I am telling you that the rules we have in place are to help you develop safely."

Consent Is About Yes (ages 11+)

"Remember when you were little and you used to ask me for tickles? You would tell me you wanted tiny tickles, not big tickles? And if I tried to give you tickles, you would say, 'I don't wanna play that game'? You were practicing how to say yes and ask for the attention you want, *and* how to say 'I'm done.' You get to decide what to do with your body and when you want to do it—no one else gets to pick for you. And you get to decide if you want to keep going or if you want to stop. And when you decide in a safe way what you want to do with your body—hold hands, hug, kiss, and someday have sex— you don't have to explain why you decided to say yes or no, because you are the boss of your body."

Legal Consent (ages 12+)

This conversation is going to vary greatly depending on where you live— age-of-consent laws are different from state to state and country to country. Rather than getting into the weeds about what is *technically* legal or allowed in your area, it might be more helpful to talk to children about what the laws are trying to accomplish: making sure that people who are not able to consent are not being allowed to consent.

Are You Ready? (ages 14+)

If your peers are doing it: "I heard that someone in your class is pregnant. That's a lot to think about—that's going to be a big change for them. It certainly makes you think about how pregnancy might impact your life. You know that pregnancy isn't guaranteed when people have sex, but when sperm and eggs are involved, it's almost always possible, even when you're careful. We haven't ever told you how long you *have to* wait to have sex—other than to make sure you knew your brain and body weren't ready as you were starting puberty—but thinking about how long you might *want* to wait is definitely something you should be doing as you get closer to getting into more serious relationships."

"I want to remind you that if you *do* decide to have sex, you can and should come to me to make sure you're using effective contraceptives. Birth control—whether condoms, the pill, an implant, or another device—is always important to use. You also need to remember that preventing pregnancy is not the only reason to use protection—you also want to prevent sexually transmitted infections. So if you need protection, or need help changing the kind of protection you're using, please come to me, or another safe adult."

The myth of tacit permission: "It might feel like by talking about sex with me that I'll 'give you permission' at some point, but I can't do that—I don't get to make choices about your body that way. Only you get to make that choice. But if you feel like I can or should give you permission to have sex, do you think you're ready yet? Part of knowing that you're ready to have sex is feeling like you don't have to explain it to me or anyone else—when you're ready, you should feel empowered and confident in the choice."

If there is any risk of later doubt, should you do it?: "Oh man, Mack looked really bummed—did he and Brandon break up? Oh, they didn't? What's up—I mean, if you want to talk about it. Do you want a Free Pass? Sure, I won't bring it up after tonight. Oh boy . . . they had sex, and now he's feeling like it was a mistake? That's really hard—was there consent? There was? Okay, well that's good. But he feels like things are different? Oofda. That's really hard. What are you thinking about it? Oh jeez, dude, 'mess around and find out' isn't super compassionate, but like . . . their situation definitely highlights how you have to be pretty confident before you jump all the way in with someone. There can be some complicated emotions afterward, but we definitely don't want doubt or regret to be in the mix. Alrighty, well, I won't bring this situation up again, but you can talk to me anytime."

What Is Rape? (ages 12+)

"Hey, we've talked a bit about what consent is, and how to know when you're ready to share your body with another person. I hope that you are only ever in situations where you feel confident advocating for yourself and that the person you're with listens to you. It's important that you know, though, that there are some people who may not listen, and who may feel like they can force you into having sexual contact with them. That is *never* okay, and there's a name for forced sexual contact—it's called rape, and it's illegal."

What Is Coercion? (ages 13+)

"Just like the F in FRIES tells us, when we give our 'yes,' it must be freely given—it has to be because we really want to. That means there can't be any coercion. To coerce someone into doing something means convincing the person to do it even though they don't *really* want to. With sex, coercion doesn't usually mean physical force—physically forcing sex is called rape, full stop. Coercion looks like mental and emotional manipulation instead."

"I was reading that book you left on the coffee table, and wow, that main character really is a piece of work. He tried to coerce his girlfriend into sex! Remember when we talked about what counts as coercion—statements like 'I'll leave you,' 'I'll be sad,' 'I won't love you,' 'Don't you love me?' 'You're a shitty partner because you don't care about my needs,' and 'I'll get my needs met by sleeping with someone else since you won't do it,' or behaviors like becoming aggressive, the silent treatment, pouting, intentionally trying to bait someone by contacting 'alternative options,' or overtly flirting with people outside the relationship in retaliation—basically, any way a person can try to manipulate another person into having sexual contact with them, that's coercion. And now I want to finish your book to see if that ever gets addressed!"

Sexual Contact Is Never, Ever, Ever "Owed" (ages 14+)

"I don't care how nice Joe is to her, Beck doesn't owe him her body. He can be as attentive as he wants and do all the 'right' things—those are *his* choices. They don't buy him sex or affection or anything. If he feels like he's putting too much in and not getting enough back, then he can break up with her. There is literally no scenario where sex is 'owed,' and if someone tries to tell you that you owe them sex—feel free to educate them. Or end things with them. Yikes."

Sometimes Sex Can Be a Waste (ages 14+)

"Man, these ads are unhinged. They put so much pressure on sex and how things 'should' be. Sometimes sex is just . . . fine. Don't get me wrong, sex can be really good, but sometimes people have sex and it isn't what they hoped, or it wasn't as fulfilling as they wanted it to be, or maybe they didn't really want to do it after all, even though they thought they did. Regretting sex happens, and it doesn't mean you or your partner did anything wrong, necessarily—it means that you both need to reassess before you try again, *if* you try again with that person."

Remember: We're All in This Together, and Lots of Us Are Lost

Acknowledging the spectrum of relationships and how people choose to engage in sexual encounters is one of the most complicated topics we'll have to discuss with our children. How do we go from discussing that consent needs to be an explicit and enthusiastic "yes" to acknowledging that some folks want an element of "cat and mouse" in their sexual encounters? Even we, as adults, don't always get the nuances correct, so how can we possibly teach our kids?

The answer is to Keep. Talking. About. It. Be honest with them—at the beginning of their escapades into romance, dating, and sexuality, there should be *no* ambiguity. "May I hold your hand?" is a great question, and even if as an adult you feel like you can read people's body language, it's not a question we should sneer at. As people get older, timing, body language, expectations, stigma, and setting all matter even more than they ever have, and are influenced heavily by the culture in which the people live. In the US alone there are a myriad of different expectations for courtship, dating, and relationships.

Unfortunately, the variability in these conversations means fitting them all into this book is impossible—there are just too many different scenarios, individual personalities, and desired outcomes to be able to spell them all out without writing an additional volume. What I *can* say is that we should continually remind our kids that their boundaries matter, that they *also* need to pay attention to the boundaries of the people they are interested in, that there will be times when they zig when they should have zagged, and that ultimately, so long as they do not hurt anyone, they will be all right, even if they are temporarily embarrassed.

Beyond navigating the complexities of establishing sexual relationships, it's also important that we discuss the other dynamics of adult relationships that kids are learning about. When I think back to the information I had access to as an early teen, I remember the most "out there" representations of sex and relationships coming from a stolen *Playboy* magazine and a couple of bodice-ripper romance novels. When I scroll the internet now, it is instantly obvious that kids have *so much more* shown to them than I ever did. I didn't even know the definition of BDSM when I was thirteen; now there are incredibly popular and painfully inaccurate fanfics, novels, and videos readily available only a click away. Even if it squicks us out, we *have* to consider that if we don't address the facts of sex and relationships with our kids, someone else might feed them full of . . . well, bullshit.

Do You Have a Condom?

This next set of scripts is very similar to scripts you'll see in the next chapter, on topics including discussions of safer sex, the importance of condoms, the need to advocate for yourself with a partner, and informed consent. As with most other topics, the dialogue around safer sex needs to be ongoing, open, honest, and nonjudgmental. The difference between those previous scripts and the following are that these next few scripts can provide ammunition for your child to use with a partner who may not be adhering to the standards your child has established for themselves.

> "Protection should not be coy—knowing how you and your partner plan to be safe is a feature of the 'Informed' part of the FRIES framework for consent. Birth control—the pill, an implant, whatever—is fine, but it doesn't prevent STIs. If

you haven't discussed each other's testing status, is that truly informed consent? You get to decide what level of confirmation you need—for some folks, just their partner's word is enough, while others want receipts—but there needs to at least be a discussion about it. You can also change your mind if your partner doesn't respect your protection needs."

"You know how I feel about condoms—you should always have your own that have been stored correctly—and if that's not okay with your partner, then y'all need to go buy them together. It can be a compromise to go get them together, but using someone else's musty, dusty, stored-in-the-glovebox-and-maybe-full-of-holes condom is not it."

"Darlin', if they are fighting with you about protection— ESPECIALLY if they are arguing that what they are doing is enough when the science says it clearly *isn't* . . . please see that for the red flag it is! The rhythm method and pulling out are not adequate protection. You know that!"

Communication Is Key—That's Why It's a Pillar (ages 14+)

"So, duh, consent has to happen before sex. But is that the only time you need it? NO. Correct. Consent is something that is super tied to communication—one of the four Pillars of Safe Sex. Remember, the *S* in FRIES tells you that consent needs to be specific. If anything changes about what two partners are doing, then consent needs to be verified—check-ins have to happen! 'Oh, we moved from the couch to my room—how are you feeling? Is this still good?' or maybe your partner wants to roll over and try another position—don't roll your eyes, this is important!—you can verify consent *and* keep it sexy. Even just letting your partner know that you like it and want to keep going is an important part of communication and consent!"

You Have a Free Pass (ages 13+)

Something to remember is that the Free Pass counts within specific discussions of sex, too. If something happens and your child feels complicated about it, or feels like it was a mistake, or wants to talk about it but not have to hear about it later—they can use their Free Pass within the boundaries you've established. So long as it's not something that will have serious long-term consequences for their health or safety, you shouldn't bring it up again after the discussion. If it *will* have long-term consequences but they are looking for your help without extensive discussion about it in the moment, then they can use their Free Pass and say they want to talk about it after the current situation has been handled and they have had time to prepare.

Reminder of when a child or teen might use this card:

+ I want access to birth control options that require a doctor (the pill, an implant, IUDs, etc.).
+ I need a morning-after pill.

- I was drunk/high and had sex that I didn't plan on having.

- I think I may have been assaulted.

- We used protection but I think it might have broken.

- I had sex and it was not fun/painful/not what I expected (or they regret it after the fact).

Some of these may sound alarming and like they should not be allowed to be used with a Free Pass, but let me remind you—if they are bringing this to you with the card, that means they may already be feeling scared about it and don't want to talk about it right now. Remember, a Free Pass isn't a promise that they'll never hear about the topic again—it's a statement that you won't push them into a larger discussion in that moment. A response like "I am not going to push you to talk about this right now, and I'm very glad you came to me for help. I need you to know that we will have to talk about this later this afternoon or this evening so that we can make sure you are staying safe" both reaffirms their choice in coming to you and establishes that you will be following up to maintain their health and safety.

If your child comes to you with a Free Pass and reveals information that cannot be left alone—perhaps they admit to inappropriate sexual contact from another adult—an explanation of why the Free Pass won't work is warranted: "I'm very glad you came to me, and I know you don't want me to follow up on this, but because this is a very unsafe situation that puts you and others at risk, I need you to give me more details because I legally have to report it."

Practicing FRIES

Just like learning to ride a bike, do their math facts, or what pigments combine to make purple, kids need to practice checking in with their boundaries and flexing their consent skills. In our house, "what if" and "would you rather" are two of our favorite games: "What if you get confronted by a hungry polar bear who escaped from the zoo?" "Would you rather find a suitcase full of cash and an abandoned baby, or find a limitless credit card and get custody of a teenager you don't know?" "What if you wake up and the rest of the world has disappeared—not dead, just . . . gone?" Sometimes the answers are silly, but it's more fun when everyone involved takes the situation seriously and tries their best to problem-solve and find logical, sustainable solutions. As my kids have gotten older, I've started peppering the games with real-life scenarios that they may run into as they start to expand their social circle: "What if you're at your friend's house and their big sister busts out the beer?" "What would happen if you were at a party and you noticed someone leading a really drunk classmate of yours to a secluded room? What would you do?"

A lot of the time, the kids have to take a minute to think about what they might be tempted to do, what they should do, and what they actually *would* do. Imagine if the first time they had to wrestle with these thoughts was when they were *in the situation*. Yikes. By considering the hypothetical situation, kids have a chance to solidify their morals *and* figure out when they might need to use their Phone-a-Friend and tap in friends or a safe adult for help.

Some hypothetical scenarios for kids to reflect on might include:

+ You find out your partner wants to have safe sex.
+ You want to have sex but your partner doesn't.
+ Your partner wants to experiment but not have "full sex."
+ You are with people who are doing drugs/drinking and someone approaches you or someone you care about for sex.
+ You are hanging out with folks and the vibe starts to feel . . . off.
+ Your friends are hanging out with people who are demonstrating a lack of respect for consent.

. . . and many, many more.

Finally, I frequently remind my kids that I couldn't care less about winning a teenager popularity contest—I will always be their out.

> "Kiddo, remember that I will always be your bad guy. I don't care if your friends hate me or not. I don't care if your partner thinks I'm the stodgiest prude who's ever walked the earth. If you need to use me as an excuse or as an escape card, absolutely feel free to do so. If they say, 'Your mom will never know,' feel free to say, 'You haven't met my mom. My mom is the WORST—she knows everything and everyone.' You can absolutely throw me all the way under the bus if it helps you stay safe and feeling like your boundaries are being respected. Just remember that if you feel like you have to use me as an out because somebody is pressuring you, you might want to reevaluate that relationship."

CHAPTER 10: IN BRIEF

Consent in sexual relationships is crucial, and also nuanced. FRIES is a helpful acronym for remembering the required components for consent, which are that it is freely given, reversible, informed, enthusiastic, and specific. Teens who are embarking on a potentially sexual relationship should identify what their boundaries are regarding sexual contact, and communicate those boundaries to their partner.

Key Takeaways

· Consent applies to yes *and* no. A person has autonomy over their body and gets to decide what they will allow another person to do to them and with them.

· Age of consent varies depending on location, but the spirit of age-of-consent laws is that there are limits about who can provide consent. If there's a question of whether its legal, it's probably best to stop and think about the choice.

· People who are impaired cannot give consent—if drugs or alcohol are involved in the interaction, be careful!

· Rape (forced sexual contact) and coercion (sexual contact after manipulation) are *never* okay.

· Sex is never owed—what someone chooses to do with their body is for them to choose. Being kind to someone, paying for food or other items, and other transactions do not "buy" sex.

· Reflecting on how to handle difficult or ambiguous consent situations before encountering them may be a helpful exercise to promote positive future outcomes.

CHAPTER 11

The Five Pillars of Safe Sex

M*y body's saying let's go . . . but my heart is saying no*, Christina Aguilera crooned out of the car stereo. Sixteen-year-old Terrance and his seventeen-year-old girlfriend, Alyssa, were sitting awkwardly in the front seat of Alyssa's car. That lyric was a bit too on the nose for their current situation. They had just been making out *very* intensely when they both realized things were escalating more quickly than they expected.

"I'm just not ready."

"I know." Alyssa sighed.

"I really wanna be with you, but I need to wait."

Alyssa felt like she needed to reassure him. "I totally get that."

"I just . . . I don't want you to be upset."

"I'm not upset, Terrance—I love you."

Alyssa dropped Terrance off at his house before heading home herself. She walked in the front door to find her mom wrapped up cozy in her bathrobe baking late-night cookies in the family's brown and beige kitchen.

"Hi, Mom."

"Hi, sweetheart—what's going on? You seem down. Did something happen with you and Terrance?"

"No." Alyssa sighed, then paused before continuing. "Mom, can I talk to you without you getting mad?"

Her mom put down the hot pads she'd used to take the cookies out of the oven and gestured for Alyssa to join her at the dining room table. "Of course you can, hun. What's on your mind?"

"Terrance and I have been together for a while now—our one-year anniversary was last week."

"I know! He gave you that beautiful necklace."

"Right . . . well, we have been talking about . . . sex."

Alyssa's mom paused, then ventured cautiously, "You're not feeling pressured to do anything are you?"

"Oh God, no, Mom. Nothing like that. Actually . . ." She tried to find the right words. "Actually, I feel like I'm ready, and he's just . . . not. And I don't know what to do with that."

Her mom was a little surprised, but knew that she needed to keep the lines of communication open, rather than shutting her daughter down by telling her to "just say no."

"Well, honey, first I want to tell you that I'm proud of you for coming to me to talk about this. Sex and relationships aren't always easy, and I'm glad you're willing to let me help you with this. Second, I want to ask—what does Terrance say?"

"He says he's really attracted to me, and that he loves me and loves us together, but that he's not ready to be with me like that. He says that he wants to wait until marriage."

"And how do you feel about that?"

"I don't know if I'm going to marry Terrance—I'm seventeen! And when I talk about it like this, I feel like I could totally wait until I'm married. But when we're together and kissing and stuff . . ."

"Your body is like, 'hell yes, more of this, please'?" her mom offered.

"YES. Exactly that. And we always manage to stop, but then it just gets weird. He apologizes and I say it's not a problem and then the mood is killed and he drives me home," Alyssa said in frustration.

"Have you two talked about what happens between making out and sex?" her mom asked.

"I mean . . . sort of? I guess? What do you mean?"

Alyssa and her mom spent three more batches of cookies that evening going over the various forms of foreplay, and how Alyssa could bring the topic up with Terrance. The high school sweethearts didn't end up marrying each other—Terrance ended up breaking up with Alyssa when he left for college—but they could both say they learned a lot about themselves and relationships during their year together. They may not have known it at the time, but this was in large part because of the Five Pillars of Safe Sex.

The open line of communication Alyssa had with her parents and her willingness to apply her self-reflection to her relationship helped keep her *and* Terrance safe as they navigated their relationship. Unfortunately, some children do not have the same kind of relationship with their parents, which is why when they have questions about how to navigate a relationship issue, they seek information online.

Though I wish I could say it's common to find supportive, accurate information on the internet, I can't. If you've ever wandered onto any number of subreddits, you know that "supportive, accurate information" isn't always the top comment. That's why it's so important for parents to work toward having open, honest lines of communication with our teens—even if it makes us uncomfortable.

I am not unfamiliar with the internal war that many of us have happening inside our brains between *NO! My babies are young and innocent, and I want them to stay that way forever!* and *My children are growing into functional happy adults . . . and most functional happy adults will have sex at least once in their lifetime.* We imagine our children growing up and having families of their own, but we don't really want to think about how those families . . . happen.

Instead of asking my children to navigate the waters of dating, relationships, and sex with only the mechanics from me and whatever information they can piece together from their friends, I tried to find a better way. I reflected on my own experiences, read the literature, spoke with other educators and professionals, and landed on what I've named the Five Pillars of Safe Sex.* These concepts—confirmation, communication, protection, lubrication, and enthusiastic participation—guide the conversations I have with my children regarding how to engage in sexual activity. They are also concepts that my children can refer back to before they embark on a sexual relationship with anyone.

The pillars themselves are pretty straightforward, though the conversations for each can be complex.

> **Confirmation** is just what it sounds like—confirming with
> your partner or partners that everyone is able and willing to
> provide consent, and that the consent is present and ongoing.

---

*Originally posted on TikTok as the Four Pillars of Safe Sex.

I've been asked why I went with confirmation rather than consent as the first pillar, and both the "ongoing" and the "able to consent" parts are the reason. Confirmation acknowledges the nuances and intricacies of sexual encounters— reminding teens (and all the rest of us) that it is necessary to confirm that consent is present, even after the first "yes." It also asks our teens to think hard about whether the people involved in the encounter are able to consent—are there drugs or alcohol involved? Are both they and their partner of an age where consent is possible (both morally and in the eyes of the law)? And is there any possibility that there might be an imbalance of power that is influencing the consent—is there money, status, or positionality that might influence whether either person feels comfortable saying yes or no? As an experienced adult, I consider these features of consent automatically, but it isn't fair to ask my teen to do the same. They should not have to unconsciously or automatically assess their partner or partners for fitness. Instead, confirmation as a pillar of safe sex inherently includes communication as a necessity for sex, which is convenient, because communication is the second pillar.

Communication extends beyond confirming that everyone involved in a sexual encounter is consenting. Even though communication seems like a fairly straightforward concept, remember that some of the conversations we're expecting our children to have with their future partners can be awkward even for us as adults. Communication requires that both partners discuss their boundaries, expectations, and experience before, during, and after sex. Boundaries and expectations include what each partner needs for protection, how kink factors into the encounter, STD and STI status, and how far each person feels comfortable going. Communication additionally asks them to consider how they plan to stop themselves in the face of their own biological urges. They also need to communicate about the experience before, during, and after it happens. That means checking in—"How are you feeling?" "Is this working?" "Should this continue?" and "How was that?" are just the tip of the iceberg. Each partner can also actively express how they are experiencing things *without* being asked! Think about the sex you've had. Was there ever a time you wish you had communicated better? As adults, we know that sex doesn't have to be mind-blowing—it can be just all right. But I know I can think back to situations where better communication could have made the experience significantly more enjoyable.

Protection is exactly what it sounds like—how a person can protect their body and (and sometimes their whole future) by making informed choices about sex. Ideally, conversations around protection frame it in nonjudgmental terms of prevention—"how to keep your body safe," "how do you disclose and discuss testing status," and "how should you talk about family planning"—rather than scare tactics about the possible unintended consequences if they *don't* use protection. Believe me—most kids know that they don't *want* to get pregnant by accident or contract an STD or STI. By reminding them what they should do rather than focusing on what they don't want, we reinforce behaviors that can keep them protected. Conversations about protection should include both protection from STIs *and* protection against unplanned pregnancy, if pregnancy is possible.

Lubrication gets its own pillar, which may be a surprise for some folks. If you're uncomfortable, I totally get it. Most of us weren't ever taught how to think about lubrication or consider it for ourselves, and certainly not how to talk about it with our teenagers. But here's the thing: There are heaps of research to back up that a lot of people would benefit from including lubrication in their sex lives, and there's even more evidence showing that for non-vaginal penetrative sex, lubrication is vital. Yes, there are situations where bodies will make enough lubrication to make the experience enjoyable, and there are some people who may never have to make additional lubrication a part of their sexual experience. However, there are many other times where additional lubrication is needed, and there are more than a few instances where the type of lubrication chosen will have an impact on health and safety. We have to be talking to our kids about lubrication options, particularly because not all lubes are created equal. Instead of taking for granted that teenagers who think they may need lube will seek information for themselves, it's on us as parents to let them know that lubrication is something they should consider. Knowing the facts about what lubrication the body makes naturally, what kinds of supplemental lubrication are available, and how to safely pick a lubricant can improve outcomes for people journeying into having a sex life.

Enthusiastic participation is the final pillar of safe sex. While enthusiastic participation is considered part of consent (the *E* in FRIES), it tells our kids that *both* parties should be enjoying the experience *throughout* the experience. Just as all the pillars are rooted in the need for consistent, high-quality communication, this pillar requires that our kids not only acknowledge verbal communication, but also understand nonverbal communication. As one of my favorite teenagers once described it, "Don't just be a stiff board, and make sure your partner isn't, either." Meaning, if either person is giving physical cues that they are not enjoying the experience, a check-in (at the very least) is necessary to see how everyone involved is feeling about the encounter.

Sample Scripts

Confirmation

Early Conversation (ages 10 to 12)

"You know how we always talk about consent—how it's your body and you get to pick—well, that's true for everyone else, too. It's really important that you understand that confirmation—making sure that both you and whoever you eventually go out with are on the same page about going out and what that means. If you want to hold hands or kiss, you have to *ask*, not just assume it's okay with the other person."

Starting to Date (ages 12+)

"You might not be thinking about it yet because you're not really ready to have sex, but you need to know that the first pillar of safe sex is confirmation. What that means is confirming consent, confirming boundaries, and confirming expectations. You've seen in movies and read in books that 'foreplay' can sometimes be coy—you know, the 'hand on the wall and lift their chin' meme. But moving forward from one act, like kissing, to the next, like sex, should never be assumed."

"What is even happening with this movie? You know that you can't assume that just because you're holding hands, you can go in for the kiss. You can't assume that just because you've been kissing, you can go into full-on making out. You can't assume that making out automatically leads to heavy petting or that heavy petting leads to sex. As a couple gets further into their relationship, they can sometimes develop the ability to read each other's behaviors and understand each other's nonverbal cues. But even in long-standing relationships, sex and physical contact cannot be assumed, and are never, *ever* owed. This movie saying otherwise is wiiiiiiild."

"Confirmation also means that you can say 'Back up, I don't actually want to do this.' Even if you've had sex with the person before, you can say 'I don't want to do it again.' And just because someone had a sexual relationship with a previous partner does not mean that they owe their next partner sex. Even if you're lying there naked with a condom on, you do not have to go through with it. At any point, you can say 'Actually, you know what? I don't want to do this,' and it has to stop at that point. You can back out. Remember, consent is reversible. And one of the pillars of safe sex is *confirming* that both people want to do what they are doing for the *whole time* they are doing it. The second either person doesn't want it, the interaction stops."

Communication

Early Conversation (ages 10 to 12)

"Have you ever noticed how when me and Jack make plans to go somewhere, we always talk about how long we're going to stay? Do you know why we do that? It's because Jack doesn't love to spend a long time with people he doesn't know, and I don't really have a good sense of time. So we talk to each other about our limits and needs before we ever go out to a place that might test our boundaries. That's an important thing for people in relationships to do—check in about their boundaries and make sure they agree on how to navigate them!"

Starting to Date (ages 12+)

"Holy crap, this movie . . . what does she think he is, a mind reader? They're showing us her inner monologue so *we* know she doesn't really want to be making out with him, but he has no idea. You know that when you're dating someone, you should literally say stuff like 'Hey, before we start, I just want to tell you, like, I'm totally excited that we're together. But I want you to know that, like, I'm not comfortable doing anything more than making out.' Because asking someone else to guess, or making yourself guess about what the other person wants, is not great communication, and it doesn't lead to informed consent."

Advanced Conversation (ages 15+)

"Hey, we've talked in the past about communication with a partner, but we've never really talked about what communication specifically looks like when it comes to sexual boundaries. It can be a bit uncomfy, but it's important to think about before you ever find yourself in a situation where you need to assert those boundaries."

"It kind of sucks that communicating during sex is almost exclusively portrayed as dirty talk. Some people really like dirty talk—that can be fun for a lot of folks—but it's not for everybody. That being said, checking in and making sure that what's going on makes both parties happy is really important. Asking if the other person is doing okay, and also letting your partner know that you like what's happening are both really good ways to make sure you're communicating your needs and respecting theirs."

"Communication as it relates to sex isn't just about communicating before sex and during sex. It also extends to aftercare and facilitating cleanup, and making sure your partner has everything they need to feel safe and secure about what just happened. 'Hey, do you wanna cuddle? Do you want a snack? Do you need a drink of water? Can you please give me a wipe so that I can clean up? Do you want help changing the sheets? Do you wanna pop through the shower?' Those are all ways to check in with each other to make sure that you both feel positive and fulfilled after the interaction has ended. You can also take that time to review what went great and what maybe needs to change if you both agree there'll be a next time."

Protection

Communication about protection is also about making sure that our kids are facilitating safer sex for themselves. Some of that facilitation comes in the form of sharing their sexual knowledge with their partners, knowing that not everyone they interact with is going to have the same level of education as they do. By encouraging our kids to fully understand and feel comfortable discussing protection, they are able to pass on rules like:

1. There needs to be a new condom for every encounter—no leaving it on to use again later.
2. No sex when anyone is drunk or high because it increases the likelihood of high-risk sex practices.
3. "Only move from front to back" applies to sex, not just wiping. You should never encourage anything to enter the vagina that has already been in the anus.
4. Check the use-by dates on condoms and make sure they've been stored correctly.
5. We should be using protection for all forms of sex, not just vaginal intercourse. This includes condoms or dental dams for oral sex, and gloves for penetrative mutual masturbation.
6. If we're going to use a toy (of any sort), it needs to either have a condom on or have been washed before we use it.

Lubrication

Advanced Conversations (ages 15+ or known sexual activity)

"Hey, when you have sex for the first time, you might think it's okay to rely on the lubrication produced by arousal along with the lubrication on the condom or other protection that you use. But here's the thing: That isn't always enough. For example, anal sex should *always* involve additional lubrication. If you are going to explore lubrication for your sexual encounters, I want you to know that a water-based lube without any additional features—no warming, no tingling, no flavoring or added fragrances—is the best place to start for your own health and safety and your partner's health and safety. Please do not use oil-based lubricants, as they can break down latex condoms. And consider waiting a bit before you consider silicone lubrication, because it can stain clothes and sheets, and until you really know what you're doing, it's not always the best choice."

Enthusiastic Participation

Starting to Date (ages 12+)

"The final pillar of safe sex is enthusiastic participation. I like to think about it as the 'do you feel like you can laugh with your partner during sex?' rule. Sex should be enjoyable, the whole time, for both people involved."

Advanced Conversations (ages 15+ or known sexual activity)

"There is literally no way during sex to tell if the other person has orgasmed unless you ask them. Never assume that you are making your partner feel good. They might be making noises or faces that lead you to believe they are enjoying the experience, but the only way to know for sure is to ask for confirmation."

"Sex doesn't have to be earth-shattering. It doesn't have to be a new and amazing and mind-blowing experience every time. Sometimes sex is just for 'scratching an itch.' That being said, you should at least both be having a good time. It doesn't have to be great, but it does have to be good. And if it's not, you need to be able to talk about why."

"Hey, I've said it before and I'll say it again: Sex is not the pinnacle of the world. Sex is not the best thing there is. Sex isn't even the best part about being in a relationship. Sometimes the best satisfaction is heavy petting and reaching peaks and orgasm and not going all the way. It's so important that you're touching base with your partner and understanding your personal goals, beliefs, and values as well as theirs—making sure that you're on the same page and that as you pursue those goals together, you're both enjoying it."

"We've talked about it before—sex is never owed. But I need you to know, too, that relationships don't have to end if you decide to abstain from sex for a while. Couples can decide to take breaks from sex and adjust what they expect for physical intimacy and still maintain a romantic relationship. So long as they are on the same page and are checking in with each other, that's just as healthy a relationship as if they were still having sex."

"Okay, I get it—'do you like that?' is a trope at this point. And that's true—you don't necessarily have to ask your partner if they're enjoying themselves as an explicit question. Maybe you agree beforehand that you're going to verbalize that things are going well. 'Yes, this is good. Hey, I like that. Hey, keep that up. More of that. Do that more. Keep doing it.' Or maybe you set up a nonverbal cue to tell each other that things are going correctly—or that they're not. Maybe you say 'If I'm nodding, it means keep going.' Or 'If I touch the bedpost, I want every-thing to stop.' Think outside the box and talk to your partner about what's going to make both of you happy in the moment. I know this is kind of a weird thing to hear from your mom, but like . . . it's really important to me that you have positive sexual experiences and that both of you stay safe."

"If anyone is pushing your boundaries or resisting your boundaries before, during, or after your sexual encounter, that is a huge red flag. Remember, boundaries are about what you will accept. So if your partner is saying, 'Hey, you don't need to wear a condom. I know you like it better when you don't, and I want you to enjoy this,' and won't drop the matter even after you insist on wearing a condom, you maybe shouldn't have sex with that person."

Another part of helping our teens prepare to have safer sex is running through scenarios they may encounter as they move into the dating world. This might look like prompting them to consider how they would assert their protection boundaries in hypothetical situations. Some examples you might use to prompt them include:

- How would you react if your partner says you don't need to wear a condom because they're on birth control?
- What would you say if your partner pulled out an ancient condom from their wallet and tried to use that for sex?
- How do you establish where you want to stop, before you ever start? How can you tell your partner that you want to make out, but you won't have sex?

Even though it feels like you just read and processed roughly five thousand words instructing you on how to help your child choose to become sexually active in a safe way (because you did read roughly five thousand words), try to remember that you do not have to memorize those words. You do not have to convey them exactly as I've written them, and you do not have to adhere to all the recommendations I've made—you, as a parent, are allowed to sort out what works for you and your child and move forward with the plan that fits you and your relationship best. If that means identifying and discussing one pillar at a time—creating your own version of scaffolding for this chapter—then I hope you write me a note and let me know how it goes so I can cheer for your ingenuity. Because ultimately, the experts on the subject of your child is your child, and you.

CHAPTER 11: IN BRIEF

Some parents worry that providing accurate, age-appropriate, comprehensive sex education may result in their child feeling like they have "permission" to become sexually active. In reality, no one can provide permission to another person for what they choose to do with their body. The Five Pillars of Safe Sex were created to give parents and their teens an easy shorthand for discussing safer sex practices.

Key Takeaways

- Confirmation asserts that both parties should confirm that informed, specific consent has been freely given.

- Communication should occur before, during, and after the sexual encounter. This includes boundary setting, questions to check in, voicing of feelings and preferences, and discussion of the experience.

- Protection should be utilized for all forms of sexual contact, should protect against both pregnancy (if applicable) and sexually transmitted infections (always), and should be used/stored according to the manufacturer's directions.

- Lubrication is required in certain scenarios, but may be beneficial in most scenarios. As such, it should be discussed and agreed upon beforehand.

- Enthusiastic participation is required by both parties for the duration of the sexual contact, or contact should not be occurring. If either party wishes to revoke consent, the interaction stops immediately.

CHAPTER 12

The Number 12 Rule (Dating)

A t sixteen, I learned what a thrill it was to sit on the back of a motorcycle. My parents were not motorcycle enthusiasts—my mom has
always felt they are more risk than reward—but in the summers of
2002 and 2003, I got to experience what everyone else thought was so cool.
I had started hanging out with a group of girls from my high school I hadn't
gotten to know well before. They were nice enough—I got invited to hang out
a bit because of a mutual friend—and we used to chill behind the main street
in our tiny little town. We also spent time at our local bowling alley, walking
through the local Walmart, and just generally keeping ourselves busy.

One of the primary qualifiers of a Good Hang-Out Spot was the
people—who was going to be there? Okay, let's not pretend it was the
people in general . . . it was the guys. Which *guys* were going to be there?
Each place had its own draw: The bowling alley was a good place to find
both your local friends and possibly some cute out-of-towners. Local stores
like Walmart and the gas station had a reliable cast of characters—if you had
your eye on someone special, you could casually shop and hope they noticed
you. "Behind main" was a bit like roulette—you never knew who you were
going to get, but it was almost always interesting.

The summers of my sixteenth and seventeenth years, a trio of men in their early twenties came to town. They were best buddies, with matching crotch-rocket motorcycles in three colors—red, blue, and yellow—and they lived together, too. These three would hang out behind main, flirt with the girls, and give the *special* girls rides on their motorcycles. Never mind that most of the girls on the backs of those motorcycles were under eighteen—that didn't seem to matter.

I remember looking enviously at the girls in the group getting special attention from the Crotch Rocket Crew—I knew I didn't qualify as pretty enough. You might think that this is negative self-talk or my memory being hard on young me, but you'd be wrong. The guys in the group had stickers on the backs of the bikes that read "No Fat Chicks" and it was clear that I was much too close to their definition of fat for anyone's comfort.

I was jealous of those girls, and I'm ashamed to admit that I slut-shamed the girls who turned the Crew's heads. I was judgmental—it didn't occur to me at the time that the special attention and sexual interactions between the girls and the Crew were more than "technically" illegal. They framed it as a bullshit law that could get them in trouble, but the Crotch Rocket Crew were all well-established adults who never should have been engaging with children the way they were. But this was the early 2000s—each of us girls had been taught by various forms of media that attention from older men was the ultimate goal, and that anyone who successfully had a *"relationship"* with an older man was more mature than her peers. And as a result, I spent months feeling sad about not being "good enough," wishing yet again that I could be shorter and slimmer and up to their standards . . . until I met Brad.

Brad was even older than the Crotch Rocket Crew. He was taller than me and rode a Harley and invited me to take a spin the first time we met. He was kind to me and gave me attention, and it seemed like he was flirting with me! I tried valiantly to flirt back . . . and was *really* bad at it. It was obvious that I was inexperienced in dating and that I just desperately wanted positive attention. It felt like Brad was kind about what I knew was my own "neediness"—he kept talking to me and giving me rides and letting me know when he was going to be in town. We even kept in touch some after I moved away for my senior year, and I always checked behind main to see if he was there when I came back to my hometown.

After I met Brad, I felt like my eyes were opened to what the Crotch Rocket Crew had been up to. I knew they had been sexually active with a few of the girls, and I knew they hadn't exactly been kind to the girls when they ended things. These girls were high school juniors and seniors who all still lived with their parents, just like me, and those jerks didn't have the same level of maturity and respect as Brad, who was willing to wait for me. I was suddenly grateful that I'd never been an object of attention for them and was happy to get on with my life . . . and keep in touch with Brad.

But after I turned eighteen, I noticed a subtle shift in the tone of our conversations. While he had always been flirtatious, after I was "legal," he was much more obvious about his thoughts. He made advances and offers to hook up a couple of times, but I always declined. Not that I wasn't sexually active by that point—I had recently become so with a man I was seeing off and on—but I knew deep down that a one-night stand or casual hookup with Brad wasn't going to make me happy. Our communications became less and less frequent, and I eventually heard that he had married and settled down and was planning to start a family.

It didn't occur to me until much later—probably my late twenties—that intentionally or not, Brad had been grooming me. I had been right to think he was smarter than the Crotch Rocket Crew—he wasn't going to risk going to jail by having sex with a minor while he was in his twenties (at least not that I knew of)—but he also wasn't opposed to trying to ensure that as soon as I was no longer a minor, I would be open to the idea. You may have anecdotes similar to this one—remembering the significantly older people who may have been pursuing us for reasons we didn't fully understand. In our own eyes, we were interesting (true) and beautiful (also true) and "mature for our age" (irrelevant), but in reality, we were impressionable, probably naive, and available as conquests. But how were we to know that, especially when we didn't necessarily know the difference between dating and grooming?

I would also wager that at that time, none of us could answer the question "What is dating?" As adults, even, we fail to remember that dating doesn't start with dinners out, picnic lunches, and long walks on the beach. For our parents' generation, dating was . . . I don't know, taking each other to the sock hop or the Sadie Hawkins dance, or maybe watching drag races in an alley—any of those tropes from all those old movies. Today, there are still some communities that have very strict ideas of what courtship looks like. They have everything spelled out from the order of the dates to when you can hold hands to when you can kiss. But for a lot of us, dating has gone from a structured practice like drive-ins, dances, and early marriage, to something more amorphous. Without clear definitions and ideas of what dating should look like, teenagers are left to take their instruction from what is modeled to them in the media they consume—YA novels, television, movies, fanfic . . . you name it. And I can tell you this much: I don't want my kid doing what most of the teenagers on television and in movies are doing. Not because dating, relationships, and sex as a teen are inherently morally wrong—but because the way it's *done* in TV shows and movies is often so unnecessarily hurtful to those involved. People end up with battered hearts and, all too frequently, minds and bodies that carry the scars of these poorly executed relationships.

So how do we lead our kids into understanding what dating is really for? The first thing we have to do is understand and explicitly define *to ourselves* what dating is for. The way I have explained it is that dating is for figuring out what we like and what we don't like, what we need and what doesn't serve us, and how to spot that in people we meet. After understanding it ourselves, we are tasked with explaining that to a child who's starting to become interested in being romantically (and eventually sexually) involved with other people.

I'm sure you've heard plenty of different perspectives on when teens should be allowed to date. People are gifted onesies for their babies that say things like "heartbreaker" or "my daddy won't let me date until I'm 30" or even "my best friend is my daddy's shotgun." I remember classmates who were told they couldn't date until they turned sixteen . . . I also remember them having a boyfriend/girlfriend at thirteen and making sure their parents never found out. I was, on more than one occasion, used as a cover story so a friend could go out on a date but tell their parents they were with me. Thankfully, no parent ever called to check—my mom and dad would *not* have covered for my friends—but the possibility was there.

In part because I was a young mom myself, the memories of these experiences were fresh in my mind when I was reflecting on what my own children's dating rules might be. Based on the cognitive and physical changes I discussed earlier, I landed on what I call the Number Twelve Rule. It's fairly simple:

1. You may not date anyone until you are twelve years old. Your brain is not ready to date because it is still learning about itself and going through a lot of changes.
2. Once you start dating, your first dates will be group dates and chaperoned outings.
3. Until you are eighteen years old, there is no dating anyone who is more than twelve months older than you or twelve months younger than you.
4. Once you are eighteen, you will not date anyone under eighteen.

These "rules" are not etched in stone—they have grace and wiggle room, just like many of the rules I have as a parent. When I posted about this rule on my social media, I got loads of comments from people who had "what-ifs" to throw my way—mostly about the "don't date anyone under eighteen" clause—and there was plenty of pushback from folks who felt the rule was too restrictive.

When I was seventeen, my boyfriend was twenty-three, and now we're twenty-four and thirty-one and we're plenty happy, thanks.

What, so if they have been together since twelve and thirteen, but now the older one is eighteen, you're going to make them break up? That's ridiculous.

Girls mature faster than boys, so it's not at all weird to see a fifteen- or sixteen-year-old girl with an eighteen- or nineteen-year-old guy.

My response to these criticisms remains the same: There might be exceptions to the Number Twelve Rule, but the developmental science tells us that individual children and teens grow and mature at vastly different rates, development that can sometimes feel like it has happened overnight, and that having no more than a twelve-month age gap is a reasonable rule to start with. Explaining that to a teenager, however, might be a bit harder.

Sample Scripts

Dating and the Number Twelve Rule

Early Adolescence (ages 10 to 13)

> "I noticed you reading that YA novel we picked up the other day—were we right? Do the main characters fall in love? They do? Ohhhhh, romantic. What did they like about each other? Similar interests, huh? Yeah, that sounds about right—dating is mostly about finding people who you like, who like you, and who you can form a connection with. There's a lot more that makes a healthy relationship, but early on it's mostly about finding people who you like to spend time with!"

> "Hey, you know that you're allowed to start going on dates with people now that you're twelve. But I don't know that we've ever really talked about what dates look like when you're twelve. So here's what the rules are: You can go on group dates, like to the movies, to the park, or to the bowling alley. You know, stuff where you and your friends can hang out and there might be

somebody in that group that you're interested in. You'll do that for a while, and eventually, if you find somebody you're really excited to spend time with, you can have dates together."

"Now that you feel ready to go on dates with just your [boyfriend/girlfriend/partner], the rules are going to shift a little bit. You can go on dates, but to start they're always going to be during the day and I'll have to make sure that I know where you are and where you're going. I'll hang out in the car. Don't worry, I won't cramp your style. But I will chaperone you when you first get started, just to make sure that if either of you gets uncomfortable, you have a way out."

"As you get more used to dating and you figure out what you like and what kind of people are good for you, you'll be able to start going on dates with just the other person, but that's at least a couple of years out. I trust you to pick people who are going to be right for you, and I trust that if you pick somebody who isn't right for you, you will find the resources and support to end it in a way that's healthy."

"Your brain and your body are changing so much, even in just the span of a year, as you're growing through your teen years. Think about how you were when you were eleven. Now think about how you are today at thirteen. Are you the same person? Do you think the same things? Do you have the same goals? Do you have the same expectations or understanding of your body? No? Okay. So is it fair to ask an eleven-year-old or somebody who's fifteen to meet you where you are? No. I agree. On top of that, it's also important to know that there are rules, depending on where you live, for how much of an age gap there can be in a relationship without causing legal issues."

Later Adolescence (ages 13+)

"Hey, I heard that Sam has a new partner—is it true that it's Logan? Oh, geez. But Logan's only sixteen and Sam is eighteen. Huh. Well, I mean, you know how I would feel about it. Yeah. I would have a lot of questions about why somebody who is two years older needs to be dating somebody who's two years younger. Hey, I'm not saying they have to break up. What I *am* saying is that maybe we should think about why that relationship is what it is. If they're a good fit, that's great, but . . . how do Logan's parents feel about this? Do they know? They're keeping it a secret?! Oh my God. Okay, here's the deal. I'm not saying that a hypothetical sixteen-year-old *has* to break up with their partner when their partner turns eighteen. Especially if they've been together for a long time and the relationship is well established, then of course not. That feels unfair. But if Logan's parents don't know, that tells me that maybe Logan's parents aren't going to be cool with it. I don't know Logan's parents super well—maybe they're really controlling and unreasonable, that's possible. But if they're not cool with it, and if Sam and Logan get together and have sex, is it possible that Logan's parents could have a really big problem with it and make life harder for Sam? I mean, I don't know what the laws are here, but it's not outside the realm of possibility, in my opinion. I just hope you know that if you were either Sam *or* Logan in this situation, your partner wanting to hide it—especially from me—is a big ol' red flag. Because I'm going to love you and root for you always, so if you're lying about it . . . what does that say?"

Boundaries

Adolescence (ages 12+)

"We've talked about boundaries before, right? You know that boundaries are what you are willing to accept in a situation, right? So, like, one of my boundaries is that I don't listen to anyone calling me names. When that one nasty coworker I had used to swear at me and get in my face, I would just leave the room, right? And I would go and talk to HR, and to the boss. And when that didn't solve the problem, I left that job and got a different one. In a relationship, sometimes people think that boundaries are what you'll let your partner do. Crap like 'I won't let my boyfriend talk to other girls,' or 'I won't let my girlfriend dress like that.' Those aren't boundaries. They can do whatever they want. If you are uncomfortable, you can assess why you're uncomfortable. If you notice that your partner calls their ex every time you have a disagreement and talks to them for a long time about how frustrated they are with you, then you could say 'I will not listen to you talk negatively about me to your ex. If you choose to do that, then I will be leaving the room.' That's a boundary. And if it's something that makes you uncomfortable and something that you really don't like, then you don't have to stay in that relationship. You cannot control somebody else's behavior, but you can control how you respond to it. Sometimes boundaries are hard to figure out—emotions like jealousy and feelings like insecurity can complicate things further—but it's always going to come back to the treatment you will or will not accept, not how to control somebody else's behavior."

"Honey, why does your phone keep going off. What is going on? Wait, what do you mean it's your partner? You canceled your date, right? I mean, how did you cancel the date? You didn't like, ghost them? No? You told them that your mom had the whole family go out of town. Okay, so why are they calling you repeatedly when they know you are with family? Wait, they expected you to just, what? Bail on us? Lie to me? No, no. No. No. No. No. No. No. No. No. No. No, no. See. That's not how this works. You are responsible for your actions, not their expectations. You followed through and communicated effectively what was going on, and just because they expect you to choose them over your family obligations does not mean that you are supposed to do that. No. Your actions are your responsibility. Their expectations are theirs, and you need to communicate with each other. But this behavior is alarming. You guys need to discuss boundaries."

"Hey, are you headed out on your date? Are you excited? Oh, I'm so glad. Got your phone? Fab. When are you planning on being back? Okay. That sounds great. Do you have enough cash? Well, what do you mean, you're on cash? They invited you, so they're gonna pay? Umm, was that something you guys talked about? No. Okay, so here's the scoop, sweetheart. You should never go on a date without any money of your own. Unless you've explicitly discussed it, you cannot assume that your date is going to buy or pay for anything for you, and you shouldn't expect that. That's not fair. I know, I know, that's rich coming from your mom. Once upon a time, I used to go on dates where I didn't have enough money to buy myself dinner. But I regret that. I feel really embarrassed by that, and I really think that that was an unfair expectation to put .on the people I went on dates with. That's part of why I want to make sure that you don't carry that through. Even though that's sometimes an expectation that we see represented in media and the way that other people talk about dating, that's not a value that we have. You should never go on a date broke, because what happens if you do and your date leaves halfway through? What are you gonna do then? How are you gonna pay for your half, or all of it? Nah, dude. If you need cash for your date, I'll get some for you."

Making Mistakes and Putting Yourself Out There

I'll never forget the first time I tried to roller-skate. I looked like a newborn baby giraffe. For some reason, I can Rollerblade like a champ, but you put those four wheels in pairs underneath my feet and I am an absolute disaster. It doesn't matter that I am fairly kinesthetically aware and have reasonable balance, or that I have practice on other forms of wheels. For some reason, me and roller skates just don't work. If I want to get better at it, I could continue to practice, but I've decided it's not a priority, and that's okay.

Here's the thing: No teenager is going to start dating and be good at it. They're all going to make mistakes. The teen years are a great time for kids to make mistakes and screw up. It's the time when they can be cringey, when they can date people who just aren't a good fit, when they can plan dates that just don't pan out. In the teen years, the stakes are generally pretty low; they still have a good support system, and as long as they have good boundaries and are making reasonable, safe choices, the consequences are relatively minimal. It's a great time to go out and screw up. So do that, please.

Adolescence (ages 12+)

> "Go on dates, try things out, see what works for you. That way, when you get to adulthood you can say 'Nah, bro, I'm not going to date people who are only into sunrise walks on the beach because I'm not a morning person and that just doesn't work for me.' You know what you like, what you need, and what works for you, and you don't waste any of your time trying to fit yourself into places that aren't meant for you."

"One of the things that's really unfortunate is that so much of our success in life is measured using a metric of permanency. In other words, permanent is the goal. We look at situations that have ended—jobs, or relationships, or friendships—and think 'Man, it would have been nice if that had been a successful relationship.' But in reality, they *were* successful situations, they just didn't last forever. I had a very successful job that lasted for eleven years—I outgrew the job. It doesn't mean that the job was not successful, I just grew past it. The same thing goes for relationships. You can have partners who are lovely and who teach you a lot, and relationships that are good while they last but aren't made to last forever. Unfortunately, a lot of the time the narratives that happen afterward are that the other person was crazy or that there was something wrong with them, when in reality, the relationship just wasn't built to last, and that's okay. So long as everyone is safe, the next priority is making sure that you can break up without hurting people. How do you break up without hurting people? Well, the same way we think about starting relationships—with communication and understanding. Never aiming to hurt the other person's feelings, never throwing them under the bus or dragging them, especially for things they can't change. There is no such thing as 'brutal honesty,' because honesty isn't meant to be hurtful. If you are using honesty to hurt someone, then you're not being honest—you're just being an asshole. *Now*, if the reason you're breaking up with them is because they're actively harmful to *you*, then the only thing I want you to worry about is ending the relationship and staying safe. Do that however you need to, and involve anyone who you need to keep you safe, including me."

When You Feel Like You Can't Do It

When you don't necessarily feel like you fit anywhere, it can be really difficult to convince yourself that relationships are worth having. You worry that all you're going to feel is rejection and that you're just going to feel like you don't fit. But here's the deal: Relationships—both romantic and platonic—are worth trying even if all you learn from them for a while is what you don't want. And while it is perfectly acceptable to opt out of dating entirely—you do not need to be partnered to be happy—making connections and finding sources of social support is vital to ongoing resilience. If you don't see the world the same way as everybody else does, it can be really hard to find good ways to hang out. My mom understood this back in the 1980s and '90s, which is why we were the house where all the kids were—kids holding Dungeons & Dragons sessions, kids playing basketball, and many a kid doing a science or English project. My mom supported my siblings and me in making friends however we could, even when we didn't fit in quite right. Being a neurodivergent person myself, I fully understand what it's like to have a brain that doesn't always mesh well with others. That's why I feel like situations that are prescribed—where there's a somewhat agreed-upon series of events, like prom—are often really helpful for kids who don't feel comfortable putting themselves out there to make friends or date. We know that a teenager's *entire* life should not be online, and they shouldn't be isolated, either. Helping our kids foster at least a small in-person community is super valuable for them as they grow, even if that means facilitating activities that we fully do not understand, like tabletop game nights, bird-watching outings, or manga book clubs.

Adolescence (ages 15+)

"Not everybody dates in high school, and that's totally fine. But making real-world contact with real-world people at the very minimum is important for your brain development for the rest of your life. Is there a club, activity, or group you might want to try to see if you can meet some folks you get along with? I'll happily make arrangements to get you there."

"I hope you know that you don't need a partner. I mean, it feels a little bit obvious, 'cause, you know, I don't have a partner. And neither does your aunt. But it's important to me that you know that it's really valuable to surround yourself with relationships that aren't romantic. There's a lot of value in having people who have your back, outside of and in addition to a romantic relationship. People who will drive you to surgery, people who will pick up your dogs. People who will laugh with you and make you think big ideas and support you and be a place for you to share your innermost thoughts and secrets. Surrounding yourself with people who love you because you are you is so valuable. And if a person in that group happens to be somebody that you're romantic with, great. But you don't have to have that."

CHAPTER 12: IN BRIEF

With general societal shifts away from organized courtship, and the advent of social media, dating apps, and instant forms of communication, the dating landscape looks very different than it did even when most of us parents were navigating it. Establishing a dialogue around what dating is for, how it can happen, when it can happen, and with whom provides kids with solid parameters for exploring their personal preferences and needs. The Number Twelve Rule also may help children identify when someone is attempting to lure them into an unsafe and inappropriate relationship via grooming.

Key Takeaways

- Children may not date while they are under twelve years old.

- Early dating is generally chaperoned group events, school functions, and interactions at school. Kids may begin to experiment with physical intimacy like holding hands and kissing.

- Due to developmental differences and differing legal statues, once a child has started dating, they should not date anyone more than twelve months older or twelve months younger than they are.

- No one over the age of eighteen should begin dating someone under the age of eighteen.

- Dating is not required, but socializing and developing a social support system are very important in fostering and maintaining resilience, so socializing should be encouraged and facilitated.

CHAPTER 13

"The Internet Is for Porn"
—*Avenue Q*

"I just can't freaking believe it. He's had the phone for what, six months? And he LOST IT ALREADY?" my friend Liz vented. "I got him a phone so he could call me in an emergency, and it's just gone." As a single mom, Liz has done a great job in raising her son, Jackson. He's respectful, sweet, smart, funny, and kind. He helps with the garbage without being asked. He does the dishes. He mows the lawn. He talks to her about his friends and video games and the books he loves. They are very close.

But he's also a tween boy, and he can be irresponsible. Just like any of his friends, Jackson sometimes forgets his football cleats, leaves his homework on the kitchen table, or neglects to brush his teeth. So this wasn't a huge stretch of the imagination—he lost his phone. He had apologized and had promised to earn the money to replace it. It seemed like everything was just going to move on until he had enough saved to buy a new one.

The night they chose to watch *Spider-Man: Into the Spider-Verse* was just like any other Friday Movie Night in their apartment. Liz popped the popcorn, Jackson prepped the movie, and they sat down to watch it together.

They watched as Miles was bitten by a radioactive spider. They watched as he turned into Spider-Man, developing his myriad of powers. They watched as Miles resisted telling his dad about the changes he was experiencing for fear of being rejected or shamed. They watched him struggle to do so many adult things when he was barely ready to handle being a teen. They watched Miles lean on help from Peter Parker, the original Spider-Man. A person who was only *kind of* equipped to care for him, and certainly wasn't unconditional in his love and support.

When the movie ended, they did what they always did—discuss the themes and takeaways. "Oh man, I loved the part when he crashed the trains in the supercollider!" Jackson said enthusiastically.

"Yeah, that was such cool animation! I thought Peter Parker was an interesting choice for a role model for Miles as he was learning to become Spider-Man. I wonder what he learned from having to almost . . . parent Miles," Liz asked aloud.

Jackson thought about it for a bit and suggested that maybe having to watch Miles be so responsible made Peter want to try harder.

"That's a good point," Liz said, "but is it really fair that Miles had to do all that? Like . . . what do you think would have happened if he had just told his parents what was up?"

Jackson was quiet. He didn't meet Liz's gaze when he said, "I mean . . . he was scared they would be mad."

"Well, yeah, he was scared—that's true. But do you think his mom and dad would *really* have abandoned him just because he was accidentally bitten by a spider? It wasn't his fault! I mean, would *I* ever leave you to deal with Kingpin all by yourself just because I didn't like Spider-Man?"

Jackson quietly agreed that no, his mom would never leave him high and dry, and that it would have been a much shorter movie if Miles had just asked for help. Then he declared that he was getting tired and walked himself up to bed.

Roughly a week later, Jackson approached Liz as she was making their breakfast. "Mom, I need to tell you something."

"What's up, bud?"

"I didn't lose my phone," he confessed. "I hid it."

"You hid it? Why would you hide it?"

"Because . . . I looked up some . . . bad pictures on it and I didn't know how to get them off of there and I didn't want you to be mad at me. So I hid it."

Liz had to take a second to process that information. He was only eleven—she didn't think she needed to be ready for the porn conversation quite yet, but clearly, they had arrived at a crossroads. She took a deep breath and began from the beginning.

"Oh, dude. Okay, so you have pornography on your phone and you were scared I'd be super pissed that you looked at it?"

"Yeah. And I saw some . . . scary stuff . . . and I didn't know how to close it."

"Oh jeez—scary stuff?"

"Yeah, some gifs and stuff."

It was time to have a thorough sit-down and get everything out in the open. She made them each a cup of hot cocoa, texted me to let me know she wouldn't be making it to hang out, and walked Jackson through the completely natural but sometimes terrifying maze that is curiosity in early puberty.

Nobody wants to pay for researching porn. Okay, that's not true—some people want to pay for researching porn, and may have financial motivations for doing so. Unfortunately, that means a lot of porn research is going to end up biased. When people have an agenda, the research is at risk of being swayed in whatever direction favors the financiers. Not all of it—I'll be the first to admit that some research into porn is relatively balanced—but it's difficult to find sources that do not have bias in sampling, measures, definitions . . . the list goes on. Because of this, we don't have a lot of great information on the impact of pornography today—we don't really understand what the change in access to pornography has done to us as humans because the children with so much increased access are not yet grown up. We have a little bit of an idea based on statistical usage, a small group of studies, and the variation in some of the diagnoses associated over time, but we only have best guesses as to what it all means. This is especially true for the impact of porn on teenage brains.

One thing we *do* know is that the age of first exposure to pornography has gotten younger than in previous generations in part because of the internet—studies vary, but the average age of first exposure generally lands somewhere between ten and thirteen years of age. Though it's not well studied, anecdotal reports assert that previously, people didn't generally interact with pornographic imagery until their early to mid-teens. Maybe somebody stumbled upon their dad's dirty magazine and brought it to the clubhouse for their friends to see, or snuck into the room behind the curtain at the back of the video rental place. Usually, they were more likely to have been exposed to nonsexualized images of bodies before they stumbled across pornography or erotica—case in point, my interest in the *World Book Encyclopedia* and *National Geographic* at a young age. But truly pornographic and erotic imagery wasn't something we ran into all that often in our pre-2000s middle childhoods.

As a result of this increase in access, we need to be having conversations with our children about pornography—discussing how the facts we *do* have about porn interact with our values and morals—and having them earlier than we ever expected to. How can we in good conscience tell our kids "Just don't look at it," particularly when we have evidence that sexualized human bodies have been a point of curiosity for human beings for centuries? By denying both the innate curiosity about such images and the ease of availability, we may choose to simply tell our kids "Don't look." And in so doing, we run the risk of shutting down the conversation . . . and risk having our kids seek information from less trustworthy sources. Instead, by saying "Here's an alternative that is safer for your brain," we both steer our kids away from doing what we don't want them to do and keep the lines of communication open.

I don't want my kids watching video pornography on the internet for a myriad of reasons, all of which I'm willing to spell out to them. As I said above, pornographic imagery and erotica has been around for millenia, and curiosity about these images is not a new feature of the human race. Video pornography, however, has only been around . . . well, since the advent of the video camera (though the zoetrope and other forms of "moving pictures" were probably used for viewing pornography long before that). And widespread easy access to video pornography via the internet has only been around since the early 2000s. It is partially this newness and our lack of understanding about the long-term impacts of pornography that makes me say "I don't want you interacting with this until your brain is done cooking in your skull, because we don't have a good idea of what it's doing to your development, but most signs point to it not being good for you."

Looking at pictures of other people's bodies is something that even I did as a kid—kids are curious, and kids who have new and precariously balanced sex hormones are some of the most curious. In the interest of balancing a curious brain with my responsibility of protecting that brain, I decided to start having conversations with my children about pornography early and to check in often. There's a lot of discussion and debate and discourse about porn's place in a healthy sexual relationship and sexual identity, and that is something for individuals to explore on their own. But as parents try to help children navigate the world of intimacy, romance, sexuality, and relationships, identifying pornography as something that can get in the way of a healthy relationship when engaged with the wrong way is something worth prioritizing.

Sample Scripts

Protecting Your Brain

Early Adolescence (ages 10+), or as Soon as They Have an Unmonitored Device—Whichever Is Earlier

"Hey, kiddo, your brain is going to get really curious soon. You will want to know what other people's bodies look like, and you might even look for images that show you what you're looking for. I know that idea seems weird to you now because you're not necessarily excited about it yet, but the time will come when other people's bodies are attractive to you. I want to talk about this with you before that happens, because it's important to me that you understand the boundaries we need to put in place to help keep you safe. Right now, I have safe search turned on on your tablet and I have unsafe images blurred out. Not because I don't think you should ever see them, but because I don't think your brain is ready to see them right now. I want you to build an understanding about your own body before you start understanding other people's bodies. Got it? And I want you to know that if you've already looked, I'm not mad at you and you're not in trouble. If you have, and you have questions, I am here to help—just let me know."

Middle Adolescence (ages 12 to 13)

"Hey. I know that you're probably curious about bodies. I was when I was your age, too. There are places where it's totally reasonable to look for bodies. Anatomy books. Art and sculpture. The encyclopedia. Honestly, even if you look for still images on Google, I totally get it. But please know that to me, protecting your brain means not looking at videos of people having sex. These videos set really unrealistic expectations for what love, intimacy, and sex look like, and it's really important right now that you make an accurate mental map of what sex and relationships are. So please don't look at videos of sex on the internet, because there are some things that your brain can't unsee."

"It's important to me that you know what your own boundaries are around images that you might be looking for on the internet. What are your boundaries? Some of the boundaries you might want to consider is knowing when to say 'I don't want to see that, please don't show me,' because at your age, it's not unlikely that your friends will see something they find exciting or interesting or shocking and they'll want to show you. And it's okay to say 'abso-freaking-lutely not.'"

"When I was a kid, one of the things that I had to be careful of was romance novels, because there are some books that portray romance and sex in inaccurate, misleading, and genuinely harmful ways. One of the popular genres were books referred to as 'bodice rippers' because they involved acts that weren't entirely consensual—the hero would rip the dress of the heroine while he was 'overpowering' her. These books made it seem like that was normal and expected, but we know it's not. So just be careful of your boundaries and protecting your brain, even when you're reading stuff that's exciting, because you can find some really shocking stuff on the internet and even in some books."

Pornography Is Not Real Sex

Part of the reason porn is such a problem is because it doesn't represent people as they usually are, which create so many unrealistic expectations about body type, hair, size, flexibility, and more. We see escalations in exploration and engagement with kink that are misrepresentative of the safest ways to practice the kink. As you know, kids learn by modeling, and it's not unreasonable to worry that frequent exposures to these misrepresentations and mischaracterizations of partners and sex may contribute to kids having unrealistic expectations about their partners in real life, and having unrealistic ideas of what a sexual relationship entails. On more than one occasion I've discussed with young clients how they felt their sexual encounters needed to frequently and consistently escalate. "I mean, nobody does just vanilla sex. It's not a thing, you know? That's so boring." When questioned about where this attitude came from, the answer was pretty simple: TV, other media, and porn. These young people were convinced that in order to have sex that was exciting and satisfying, they had to be acting like the actors they saw on their screens.

Viewing porn—specifically on ad-supported sites or on the dark web rather than pay sites—gives the creators traffic and potentially money. If the videos people watch are created using unethical means, that traffic and money might encourage the creators to make more. I know that I do not want myself or my children to be participating in a system that hurts people or that's actively harmful. Unfortunately, the money-and-power side of pornography isn't necessarily the first thing people think about when they get curious about sex and porn—they look first, ask questions later. By including some of these ethical dilemmas in my conversations with my children, I hope I can persuade them to understand this: Part of the reason it's really not a good idea to be looking on the internet for porn videos, particularly on ad-supported free sites or via downloads on the dark web, is that each click and each view has the potential to perpetuate human harm.

It would be naive of me to assume that encouraging my children toward still images, art, anatomy books, and similar would result in them exclusively looking at those sources. So as much as it pains me, I have included a discussion of what seem to be the least actively harmful places to look for videos, if they should find themselves curious.

Older Adolescence (ages 13+)

"Hey, we've talked before about how you should really avoid watching pornographic videos on the internet, and I want to make sure you understand why, especially now that you're starting to date. Most of the people who make those videos are not portraying sex, intimacy, and relationships accurately. Just like actors in movies we see at the theater have special effects and makeup and all kinds of stuff to make them look a certain way, people in pornography are not true representations of what most people look like naked. Beyond that, the way that sex happens in porn videos is not what sex is like in real life. Remember the Five Pillars of Safe Sex we talked about: confirmation, communication, protection, lubrication, and enthusiastic participation. They do not exist in most porn, and that's a problem, especially as you're trying to figure out what sex is *supposed* to be like."

"It might make you feel weird to talk about this, but we need to chat about why porn is a problem, beyond the fact that it's inaccurate. And not because it exists at all, but because so much of it is produced unethically. What that means is that people who are in those videos aren't always in those videos with their full consent. Sometimes the people in the videos are doing the videos because they're feeling really pressured, because they want love and approval, because they need money, or because they're addicted to drugs. In the worst cases, they don't want to be in those videos at all. It's not even coercion, it's rape. I don't want you to be watching those videos because I do not want you to be building your mental expectations of sex based on examples that do not include consent."

Curiosity, Safety, and the Law (ages 11+)

"All right, I'm letting you have a phone, and I know you're super excited about it. You've been waiting for a while, and you've done a lot to show me that you're responsible enough to have one. That being said, I want you to know there are some rules. I have the passwords to everything, and I can check your phone at any point. I will not dig super deep into what you're doing on the phone. Like, I don't need to know what you and Ashley are planning every night or talking about, or the bands you're into. I trust that you'll share with me what you want to share with me. But I do need to know that you're making safe choices about what you share with other people. And I need to know that people aren't sending you things that are not good for your brain. These rules will relax as you get older, but as a new phone user, it can be really tempting to do things that are against what you know to be right. And these devices are made to be addictive and to, like, bait you into doing stuff. So I'll help you learn how to use it, and as you show me that you're making good choices, we'll revisit the rules. Sound good?"

"Hey, nerd, is there anything you can do to make me stop loving you? No. You're right. There's nothing you can do to make me stop loving you. I'm saying that because I want to remind you that if you see something on the internet, like if you're looking for stuff and you see something that scares you, I want you to know that you can and should tell me. I'm here to be your safe grown-up, and to help you process things that freak you out. I can't help you if I don't know it happened. So you can absolutely come to me and tell me if you've seen something that scares you, and I promise you will not get in trouble. We might have to make adjustments to boundaries, but you're not going to get punished."

"Hey, kid—pop quiz! The internet is what? Forever. Correct. What does that mean? Yes, it means that you should not put things on the internet that you wouldn't want your Nana to read, because Future You will probably be very upset that Past You put them on the internet. It also means that you need to be really thoughtful about what you take pictures of and what you share with people. Because here's the deal: Naked pictures of your body are considered child pornography, and that's *illegal*. They should not exist on your phone or anyone else's phone, even if you took them and sent them to your partner who is the same age as you."

"Reminder—if someone sends you pictures of themselves naked, or somebody else naked, I need you to let me know immediately. Seriously—any pictures, videos ... any naked or nearly naked bodies at all. It's illegal when you're a minor. I know it might be tempting to share pictures of your body, and when you become an adult that will be your business. But you and your friends are minors—pictures of y'all in any state of undress are literally illegal. Further, if people are sending you pictures of *someone else*, that's super questionable, because that other person likely didn't consent and there may be some legal ramifications for sending the picture. There are laws and rules and ethics about all of this, and I want you to tell me if anything like this ever happens because it would be unfair and wrong of me to ask you to figure out how to handle that on your own."

What *Is* Grooming, Anyway? (ages 12+)

"Dude, I get it. You're angry with me. Your friends have social media and you don't. Firstly, you are not thirteen yet, and the terms of service for all of those apps require you to be thirteen. So it might feel like I'm the buzzkill, but it's not just me. Secondly, there is a reason why I will be helping you learn how to use social media when you are allowed to get it, and it's the same reason I make sure I get to know all of your teachers and why I am the one on the team contact app. As you get older, you might run into older teens and adults who find you attractive even though they know and you know that you are too young to 'be with' them. So instead of asking you out or making it clear that they want to get into a relationship with you, they will start by asking you to do them favors, asking you to keep secrets, and asking you to do things that make it seem like you have a special status. And then they can use the relationship they've built with you to manipulate you into doing things with them that are not appropriate for a kid your age. People who do this are very, very good at it, and it would be unfair for me, as your mom, to expect you to avoid people like this without first learning how to. So when you start on social media and branch out into social settings by yourself, we'll keep touching base and talking about who you are hanging out with, who is sending you messages, and all that stuff. And after a while, you'll start to get a gut feeling about what feels right and what might be sus—and act accordingly! And finally—your digital footprint will follow you around *forever*. I promise you'll thank me when you have fewer cringey old posts following you around than your friends do."

Curiosity and Self-Esteem

Adolescence (ages 12+)

"It's not a bad thing for you to be curious about bodies. No, it doesn't make you gross. It doesn't make you impure. It doesn't mean there's something wrong with you or that you're a slut. It just means you're curious. There are lots of different opinions about curiosity and about bodies, but I need you to know this: I know that you're curious, and that's okay. There are safe places to look to learn about sex and intimacy and bodies."

"Your curiosity does not label you. Wondering what another person's body looks like, or needing to know the definition of a term does not mean you suddenly have a label attached to you based on your curiosity. If you want to see pictures of other people's bodies who happen to be the same sex as you, that's okay—it's normal to be curious. Just because you want to understand what a term you read means does not mean that you want to do it. Just know that curiosity and identity are not the same thing, and curiosity does not dictate who you are."

The Spank Bank (13+)

It has come to my attention that not *everyone* has seen the classic 1999 film *10 Things I Hate About You*, and as such, do not have a frame of reference for the term "spank bank." In the film, a character is trying to dissuade his friend from pining after a girl. He tells the lust-struck young man that he has no shot with the very popular young woman and says, "Add her to your spank bank and move on."

People often use pictures, movie scenes, fine art, literature, and mental images of other people as inspiration during self-pleasure. A "spank bank" is a repository of tried-and-true, go-to mental (and sometimes physical) images that an individual can access in private for such inspiration, rather than having to seek new inspiration every time.

As a counselor of young people, I have come to very much appreciate the idea of a spank bank. One of the most concerning trends I have seen in recent years is both the rate of porn addiction in young people, and the escalation of porn search themes and topics. As I was researching how to deal with this for both my clients and my own children, I was reminded of the concept of a spank bank. Though it might seem counterintuitive for a parent to explain what a spank bank is or encourage their child to have one, the logic is straightforward—better to tell your kid that you know they might be using inspiration and offer guidelines than have them end up seeking questionable, escalating inspiration online. And I'm not the only person who has thought of this—while writing this book, I asked a friend if she knew the term "spank bank" and she replied, "Oh yeah, I'm pretty sure I've heard Eric [her husband] talking about that with Luke [her teenage son]. We'd rather he have some go-tos than end up on PornHub or something."

> "Hey, do you know what he means by 'spank bank'? Okay. So you get it that a spank bank is basically a group of tried-and-true images or inspiration for someone to masturbate to. Okay, listen. Here's the thing. It's totally normal to be turned on by other people's bodies, right? That's a thing we've talked about, and it's also totally normal to have specific things that do it for you. And here's the deal. If there's a particular scene in a movie or portion of a book or image that you've seen in a magazine that really revs your engine, go ahead and turn it on.

People use 'inspiration' like pictures, movie scenes, and porn to masturbate, and they have since time immemorial. If I'm not home, if I'm out shopping and you want to pop in the DVD to watch that one scene from that one movie . . . like, just . . . all I ask is that you lock the door so I don't walk in on anything. I don't think that's weird or wrong. It's totally okay, and having those kinds of things in your back pocket can protect you from looking for new and exciting things that may not be in your best interest. Okay, fine. I promise I won't bring this up again while we finish the movie. Just know that that's where I stand."

How to Help When They (Inevitably) Screw Up (ages 12+)

As parents, we need to consider how we're going to handle our children's panic when they screw up, because our kids are *going* to screw up. They're going to see things they didn't intend to look at; they're going to search for things we wish they wouldn't; and even if they don't actively look for it, they might stumble upon things that gross both of us out and make us feel weird. I am of the opinion that we have to decide how we're going to handle it before this happens, because allowing our emotions to get the better of us in the moment is often where we end up unintentionally doing damage to the relationship. Much like the story that began this chapter, we have to think about what we're going to do when our kids feel like they've done something unforgivable. The answer, of course, is that any response must remind them they are always worthy of our love and compassion and grace, and then help them figure out how to rectify what they may have done.

Something even scarier is the possibility that the mistake made might include our child finding something that is actively harmful to the person in the photo, post, or video they've seen. How do we handle it if our child interacts with something that is legitimately illegal and reportable to the authorities? How do we respond to that? How do we know that our children will even come to us if that happens? The best way I can think of is to address it head-on, to say to our children flat out:

> "If you see something where someone is being harmed, even if you're worried that I'm going to be mad about it, I need you to tell me. Because the only way that we can keep your brain safe and try to prevent harm coming to people is if we can report what we found. There are people whose whole job is to try to shut down people who are harming others. And if we can be part of that by reporting things we see that we know are wrong, then that's what we can do to help. Even if you're worried that I'm going to be upset that you were on the wrong side of the internet, even if you have to disclose to me that you were downloading things when we talked about you not doing that, even if you're worried that I'm going to judge your preferences, I need you to know that none of that will come before me saying thank you for trying to keep people safe. Let's deal with the problem at hand. I will never stop loving you, even if the mistake you made feels huge."

CHAPTER 13: IN BRIEF

Curiosity about the human form and the use of imagery like sculptures, paintings, and eventually photographs for sexual stimulation have been part of human life for centuries. Acknowledging this fact of our existence and determining how to navigate the recent boom in the availability of pornographic images and videos is one of the more difficult tasks parents face. There is not a lot of research on the impact of pornography on developing brains, so I propose a moderate approach.

Key Takeaways

- Curiosity is normal and is nothing to be ashamed of. However, curiosity should be guided into outlets that have a longer, slightly more researched history, like still images, art, and literature.

- The internet is full of information—some of it is helpful, a large part of it is not. Please think before you click and take most results with a grain of salt.

- The internet is also *forever*—children should be restricted from creating online personas and social media accounts until they can cognitively grapple with the abstract idea of a digital footprint.

- Pornographic videos do not depict real human relationships, and many available for free online are produced unethically—children should avoid them for the safety of their brain development.

- If a child admits to having viewed pornography or to seeking it out, parents should react compassionately while also setting boundaries to protect their child's developing brain.

CHAPTER 14

Pride

I didn't figure out how tiny my world really was until I attended All State Choir. The town where I grew up wasn't exactly diverse. Beyond the representation I saw on TV, my world was very straight and white. That didn't change until I went to All State Choir camp, where I was introduced to other kids my age from all walks of life, some of whom were openly gay. The way in which this expanded my world was one of the highlights of the experience, and I'm grateful that my children are growing up at a time when more people feel able to live as their authentic selves.

But we still have a long way to go toward equal representation and universal acceptance. It can be hard to move away from heteronormative speech and into discussing what might be an uncomfortable topic for you as a parent, especially if your values do not align with non-heteronormative ways of living. I acknowledge this difficulty, and I applaud your willingness to engage with the challenge. If you are struggling—if you are feeling like you shouldn't discuss these topics with your children as they grow—please consider this: When you get to the heart of the issue, your children's safety, and sexual safety in particular, is much more important than your potential discomfort at having to answer questions about a community to which you don't belong, or about a lifestyle with which you may not agree.

Before we go too far, it's important that we discuss some definitions and clarify some concepts so that everything we discuss going forward is understandable and correct—and so that you can address these subjects confidently with your children.

> **Biological sex** generally refers to the physical sex characteristics present on an individual, most commonly primary sex characteristics like a penis or vagina. Biological sex exists on a spectrum that is influenced by factors including genetics, fetal development, and hormones. The sexes I will refer to are male (having a penis), female (having a vagina), and intersex (having ambiguous physical sex characteristics).

> **Gender** refers to the socially constructed characteristics attributed to masculinity and femininity. In other words, gender is the collection of attributes that determine if someone is a "woman" or a "man." Gender is typically assigned to an individual at birth depending on what external primary sex characteristics they possess.

> **Gender identity** is an individual's own understanding of their gender, and its relationship with their culture's expectations of masculinity and femininity, as well as the labels (man, woman, nonbinary, agender) attributed to each.

Gender expression is the outward representation of gender. This includes physical attributes like clothing, hairstyle, and accessories, as well as other forms of expression like voice modulation and pitch, behavior, name, pronouns, and other factors that may or may not align with societal definitions of masculinity and femininity.

Trans, as in transperson, transgender person, transwoman, or transman, refers to an individual whose gender identity does not align with the gender they were assigned at birth. They may or may not choose to outwardly transition their external gender expression to match their internal gender identity.

Sexuality refers to an individual's place on the spectrum of sexual attraction. There are several clinical and research scales that can help categorize where people may fall on this spectrum, but some of the identities include straight (attracted to the opposite sex), gay (attracted to the same sex), lesbian (attracted to the same sex; specific to women), bisexual or pansexual (attracted to individuals irrespective of their gender or sex), and asexual (no sexual attraction).

I wish I had the space in this book to fully answer all the questions you and your kids might have about LGBTQ+ topics, but the reality is that I do not. There are too many nuances and complexities in the world of human development for me to be able to do them justice. Instead of trying to jam little bits and pieces into paragraphs and fail to get enough accurate information to you, I have provided a list of books, websites, and other resources in the back of this book (see page 285).

What I can cover in this book are some of the more common topics that may come up with all children, regardless of identity. If you have to choose between asking your child to fend for themselves with the potentially questionable information they are able to find on their own and providing your child with information that keeps them safe, you're going to pick safety every time. Even if it makes you uncomfortable. Even if it means your child may not share your values. Even if it means seeking out answers to questions you never wanted to ask—your primary goal is to make sure they have the information that will help them be safe. Because this safety is not just about their development—it's their life, and the research out there already shows this. A study published in the journal *Pediatrics* found that lesbian, gay, and bisexual children who were rejected by their families were 8.4 times more likely to have attempted suicide, 5.9 times more likely to report high levels of depression, and 3.4 times more likely to use illegal drugs.

I want to be very, very clear: You may think that gay people should not be allowed to get married. You might feel like transgender people are crazy. In the context of this book, none of that matters. You are your child's first teacher—about life, about love, and about family. You have the opportunity to model empathy, compassion, and a willingness to learn. Furthermore, by demonstrating a willingness and exercising your responsibility to see your child's humanity first and foremost, you may be improving their overall health outcomes. Family acceptance has been found to be a protective factor for LGBTQ+ youth, and predicts greater self-esteem, social support, and generally positive health outcomes. This may be additionally beneficial to LGBTQ+ youth who are bullied at school about their identity, as they have been found to have higher rates of negative health outcomes in adulthood.

Learning how to find community can be really difficult for kids, especially as they're navigating their identity. Knowing who to reach out to for support or where to ask questions can be particularly hard for kids who were not raised surrounded by representation or with people in their close inner circle who also belonged to the LGBTQ+ community. Cultural ideas like slang, rules and norms, and how to navigate the social aspects of their identity are generally only taught by people within the community. One of the things we as parents can do is figure out how to create community for our kids. Seeking out organizations that support LGBTQ+ kids as well as their families and allies is a great first step in building this community for our children and for ourselves (see the resources section on page 285 for some recommendations).

For our kids' entire lives, they will see us for who we are and recognize our morals and values in our actions. This is great when we're trying to model our beliefs and help our children make choices that we think will benefit them over the course of their lives. However, it can also be a double-edged sword, especially if we've let our children see things that make them feel invalidated or unsafe. What I mean is, how do we do mitigate the damage if we've done or said homophobic, transphobic, or other harmful things in front of our child who identifies as gay, or trans, or otherwise feels hurt by what we've done? How do we show them that we are safe if we've previously demonstrated unsafe behavior? How do we bring back unconditional positive regard if we've shown that in some situations, our positive regard is actually . . . conditional? I believe the first step, as with everything, is communication: acknowledging the mistake we made, identifying with our child what they may have internalized from witnessing the mistake, and reestablishing the truth of our unconditional love and unconditional positive regard. Acknowledging a mistake in this way is a skill that many people struggle with—I've heard it from lots of clients: Knowing how to apologize is something they don't have a lot of practice with, and it can be incredibly hard to find the words, especially when the mistake was an expression of a core belief.

As we venture into these sample scripts, please remember that we are doing so with our Foundation of Unconditional Positive Regard, and our respect for Curiosity and Consent for Knowledge centered in our minds.

Sample Scripts:
Early Adolescence (ages 10 to 13)

Identity Exploration (ages 10+)

As parents, it might be difficult to remember what middle school identity panic felt like. We feel so comfortable in who we are as grown-ups that we forget how difficult it was to figure out where we fit when we were preteens or teenagers. When our children are going through the period of life where they're trying to figure out where they fit, they may try on identities that we know nothing about. Some folks may feel the need to react in some specific or strong way, while other folks may react without thinking at all. Identity development is a complex, nuanced, important topic that cannot be covered in one conversation, but the Foundations of Unconditional Positive Regard and Curiosity both come in handy when discussing identity with growing children. What I can also say from professional experience is that children are likely to cycle through several different versions of themselves before they begin to feel comfortable in who they are.

As you read earlier, the best outcomes for all kids occur when they are developing in a supportive environment where they feel safe and accepted for who they are. For parents who do not belong to the LGBTQ+ community and for parents who view themselves as allies, it's important to consider how you might handle your child processing their identity exploration with you and how you might handle it if they come out to you, before it ever happens. It's also valuable to be familiar with the definitions covered earlier in this chapter and prepared to define them for your children.

> "Hey, I've noticed you've been a little bit quiet lately and you've switched up your look quite a bit, is something going on? No? Okay. Well, I just wanted to remind you that, like, at this stage of your life, it's okay to be unsure of who you are and what you think about things. And I'm going to love you regardless. Remember, labels are for soup cans. Right now in your life, you're figuring out who you are and figuring out what you like and what makes you feel good emotionally and physically. It's okay to not be sure about anything right yet. I love you, forever and always. You can be flexible and make discoveries about yourself for as long as you live, and nothing is going to change how I feel about you or how any of the people who love you feel about you, okay? So you don't need to feel like you need to label yourself or give me any sort of

definition. Or announce to the world anything about yourself until you're ready, and maybe even not ever. And if you *do* decide on a label, I am happy to know about it when you're ready to share it. Okay? Okay. I just wanted you to know."

"I need you to know that you don't owe anybody your story. We've talked before about how labels are for soup cans, and that you don't have to even have a label for yourself. But I also want you to know that if you've decided on a label, you don't owe anybody to share it. You get to decide what your level of privacy is and how you want to live your life. We've seen a lot of stories about how people 'came out of the closet.' Those folks coming out and being open with their lives—that's super great for them. I'm proud of people who feel that that's the best choice for them, and I will be proud of you, too, if that's the choice you make. But I want you to know that you don't have to do that until you're ready, and maybe not even ever. There are people who choose to keep their lives private, and you're allowed to do that. You're also allowed to tell only some people, or to tell everyone—your story is yours, and I will support you in whatever choice you make."

"Thank you for choosing to come out to me. I know that can be a big step, and I'm really grateful that you decided to include me in it. I'm proud of you and I love you."

As much as we hope that our children feel like they can come out to us, we must contend with the fact that they may not. Regardless of the reason why—fear, shame, or otherwise—our children may choose to be "out" in spaces like school or with friends, but not to us. That may send you through a whole gamut of emotions, wondering why they didn't tell you first. I encourage you to process those emotions by reaching out to friends, family, and social connections who feel the same way you do about unconditional positive regard. Resist the urge to process (or even express) complicated or mixed emotions about this change to your child. They are navigating their identity expression—what they need from you is support.

> "Hey, I noticed you changed your pronouns on the school website. Would you like me to use those same pronouns? I will do my best to and I will remind our friends and family to do that if you'd like."

> "Someone asked me today if I liked your new boyfriend, and I told them I'm still getting to know him, but you seem happy. You don't *have* to tell me about him—I'm sure you have reasons why you haven't told me about him so far, and that's okay—I just want you to know that what I care about most is that you are happy and safe, not what gender your partner is."

Love Is Love

One of the more vocal arguments against representation or discussion of queer relationships is that "young children shouldn't be exposed to that." This, of course, ignores that plenty of children grow up to be queer in some way—the survey of US Census information from 2021 found that of adults age eighteen and older, 4.4 percent identify as bisexual, 3.3 percent identify as gay or lesbian, and 4 percent identify as "something else" or are unsure where they fall on the sexuality spectrum. The protest also ignores that there are children right now growing up with queer parents. As we've talked about before, acknowledging and affirming that something happens—in this case, people have sex—does not make it happen. The same applies with acknowledging and affirming queer couples—it's not going to make children queer. What it *will* do is show your children that you want people to exist in happy, healthy relationships, regardless of their identities.

I remember getting stopped by the principal of the school where my child was in kindergarten. The school had received a call from the parent of a classmate who was upset about my child. "Yeah, apparently your son and their son were playing house with another little girl. She said she wanted to be the dog instead of the mom, so your son said to the other boy that they could just both be dads of the dog. Their son came home and told his folks and they're pretty upset. It might be best to have your son keep that kind of stuff at home." I told the principal that I would not be doing that—at the time, Minnesota had just passed legislation legalizing gay marriage, and my son had several gay families in his life that he was not going to be raised to be ashamed of. I pointed this out to the principal—that gay marriage was the law of the state and likely to soon be law of the land—and to my pleasant surprise, he agreed with me. It unfortunately meant that the parents of the other little boy forbid him from playing with my son, but I hope that even that small interaction let that little boy know he didn't *have* to feel the same way.

> "Did you know that boys can marry boys and girls can marry girls? It's true! A grown-up can love any other consenting grown-up!"

"I heard someone in your school say that something they didn't like was 'gay.' And I wanted to touch base with you about it because 'gay' isn't a word to describe bad stuff—it's what a relationship is called when a man loves a man. When a woman loves a woman, they are called lesbians. Some people don't feel like they want to be in a relationship with anyone, and they're called asexual. And some people love all kinds of other people, and they're called bisexual, or pansexual. None of those words are insults or used to describe bad things, so I wanted to make sure you know what they meant."

"I wanted to touch base and make sure we are both on the same page about how growing up is going. Does that sound fair? Okay. Well, I wanted to make sure that we're both speaking the same language about bodies and identity. You know that me and your dad are a married couple, but did you know that we're what people call a straight couple? Yep! We're straight, or heterosexual, because I'm a woman and your dad is a man and we're attracted to each other. Some other couples that have two men, or two women might be called gay, or lesbian, or queer. Yup! And as you grow up, you'll figure out what kind of couple you might want to be in."

"Remember, when I say 'men' and 'women,' I mean anyone who identifies as a man or anyone who identifies as a woman. Mom's friend Eddie is a transman, but I just call him a man.

So when I talk about relationships between men and women, that includes trans folks!"

"Same-sex relationships really aren't any different than heterosexual relationships. They still involve people getting to know each other, deciding that they like and appreciate the other person and want to spend more time with them. Same-sex couples still have to talk about consent, and boundaries, and goals, and expectations, and work on establishing a healthy relationship with good communication."

Discussing Other Types of Sex (ages 10+)

"We've talked before about how sex is to make babies, and also that it feels good. Before, when we've talked about sex, we've been talking about what's called vaginal sex, or heterosexual sex. That means that one person has a penis, and one person has a vagina. For people who have the same parts—two people with a penis, or two people with a vagina—they have sex, too. The sex they have feels good for them but doesn't make babies. All kinds of sex should only happen between grown-ups who talked about their choice and have given consent to each other.

"Sometimes grown-ups put their mouths on the other person's genitals—that is called oral sex. Another kind of sex is when one grown-up puts a part of their body like their fingers or penis into the anus of another grown-up. That is called anal sex. These kinds of sex still follow the same rules—they are for consenting grown-ups who are following the Five Pillars of Safe Sex."

Later Adolescence Scripts and Reminders (ages 13 and older)

It's important to remember that the Five Pillars of Safe Sex apply to all kinds of sex and should be reviewed with children irrespective of their sexuality or gender identity. Same-sex couples may not face the same pregnancy risks that heterosexual couples do, but they still have to contend with potential health risks of sexual behavior, and still need the support of their parents in navigating their choices.

"I know you and your partner have been together a pretty long time now—I'm glad to see you so happy. I can see you cringing, but I just want to remind you—even though y'all are the same sex, you still need to be using protection when you have sex. I know, I know, you're not risking any babies. But protection is still necessary to prevent STIs."

"Reminder: The condoms are under the sink. They need to be used for any penetration—oral, vaginal, or anal. Yes, every time. The thin black box is non-latex, if that's necessary."

"Oral sex on someone with a vulva requires a dental dam. You can just take a condom, cut the tip off, then cut it lengthwise. That way the latex can be held up and make a thin barrier between the vulva and vagina and the other person's mouth. Because yes, you can still get STIs from oral sex."

On Body Dysmorphia

As you've no doubt figured out, I almost exclusively use biological terms when discussing bodies. This helps avoid confusion and helps my children advocate for themselves effectively. However, I don't believe that everyone should use biological terms exclusively. Some limited studies have found that for kids experiencing gender dysphoria or body dysmorphia, choosing to use alternative, agreed-upon names for certain body parts may be a way to ease communication and improve discomfort. For example, I may choose to opt for "chest" rather than "breasts" for a child who is questioning their gender. "Chest" is a genderless and accurate term, whereas "breasts" is generally perceived to be gendered. This mode of communication may take some getting used to and will almost certainly require advocacy from you as a caregiver when dealing with people like physicians, but for tweens and teens who are struggling to communicate, taking gender off the table entirely may be a helpful strategy.

CHAPTER 14: IN BRIEF

Moving from heteronormative discussions of sex into conversations that include the entire spectrum of sexual identities, gender identities, and romantic identities can be difficult and awkward, particularly for parents who are not part of the LGBTQ+ community, but it is a necessary part of providing children with a comprehensive picture of sex and relationships. This requires parents to educate themselves on topics that may not make them comfortable, but that can prove to be vital in their child's future.

Key Takeaways

- Family acceptance plays a huge role in the health outcomes of LGBTQ+ youth. Reiterating unconditional love and unconditional positive regard should be the first step in discussions of any topics related to LGBTQ+ identity.

- Queer relationships are not fundamentally different than straight relationships—they are based on the same factors, including intimacy, passion, communication, respect, and commitment.

- Other forms of sex, which occur in the context of same-sex *and* heterosexual relationships, including anal sex and oral sex, should be discussed with the same biological precision as vaginal sex.

- All sexual contact—same-sex, heterosexual, oral, and non-penetrative—should all be practiced within the boundaries of the Five Pillars of Safe Sex.

- When in doubt, reach out to professional organizations to help guide you and your child with accurate, compassionate, science-based information.

CHAPTER 15

Remember, Remember.

I will never forget coming home to tell my mom that I was pregnant for the first time. I was nineteen years old, living with a roommate some three hours from home. I had a very unstable work history and had dropped out of college because I couldn't balance a 17-credit course load with living off-campus and working forty hours a week. My on-again, off-again boyfriend was absolutely not going to acknowledge or support a pregnancy.

I sat her down in the great room of my childhood home. My dad had been dead for four years, and our relationship had been rocky in the aftermath—our co-occurring grief mixed with the rebelliousness of my teen years was not a great combination. I was beyond nervous—my stomach was swinging between "lava pit" and "Stonehenge" and was definitely not going to settle anytime soon. I gathered up the words . . . and promptly lost them. I had to just show her the paper from the doctor that had the undeniable results:

Pregnancy: POSITIVE

My mom took the paper from my hands, and I don't think I breathed at all while she read it. She took the information in, looked at my face and said, "Well, if this is true . . . what's the plan?"

"I'm going to keep it."

"Have you told anyone else?"

"No."

"We need to tell your sister."

My older sister was as close to a second mom as she could humanly be. She had nannied me every summer through most of my childhood and taken in my younger brother and me after my father died unexpectedly and my mother was hospitalized for several months.

I started to cry. "Mom, I can't tell her. I can't say the words to her."

"I'll tell her."

She called my sister and gave her the news. My sister was both scared for me and a bit disappointed in me (my mom was, too—they knew this wasn't going to be an easy road), but offered nothing but unconditional love, guidance, and support that made an indelible mark on my soul. Both my mom and my sister have been instrumental in the raising of my eldest child, and they were the models I used when it came time to show my children what unconditional positive regard looks like.

Writing this book, I had to identify takeaways. What did I think was the most important thing for a person reading this book to walk away remembering? And even though each chapter has its own list, the overall, whole-book list was surprisingly short. It really is only two things: 1) your child should always know that you care about them before anything else—that there's nothing they can do to make you stop loving them. And 2) presenting information to our kids doesn't *make* anything happen—it can help keep them safe. Teaching your children the facts about sex, how to look for accurate information about sex online, or the steps to being safe during sex will not make your children suddenly decide to become sexually active, or change who they are inside. Knowledge of physical health does not compromise a child's morality—all it does is give them information that can help keep them safe.

With that in mind, there are some thoughts I haven't yet shared that we need to address before we part. These are the heavy hitters—the ones that many of us will wrestle with, because they are so different from how we were raised. The cycle-breaking conversations. The "I love you and trust you to make the right choice for you" discussions. Things are way different now for teenagers than they were when we were teenagers. Social media, the internet, and lightning-quick access to both information and consequences are things we didn't have to grapple with. Before we, as parents, can have these scary conversations, we need to do a lot of self-reflection. We have to work on our own emotional regulation so that when our kids need us to be there to support them, we aren't stuck in our own feelings, or reliving our own traumas and mistakes and projecting our hurt onto their potential choices.

We also have to remember that getting hurt is part of how we grow and learn what we will and won't accept. It sucks to watch your child cry over a crappy breakup. It's almost unbearable to watch the aftermath of a relationship riddled with coercion you were powerless to stop. Our kids are going to make mistakes, and it's going to be so hard to watch them do it when we could just . . . tell them what they'll learn from it. But for some of us—myself included—the only way to learn is from experience, even if it's going to be painful. And we know that we'll be there for them while they process the finding-out.

I want you to remember that accurate information does not have to be at war with your deeply held beliefs. Your personal moral compass, your inner voice, or your faith can be unshakable, and you can still provide your kids with information to help keep them safe. Believe me when I tell you that you can believe that waiting for marriage is the best way to treat sexual activity *and* provide safe-sex information to your kids. They are not and shouldn't be mutually exclusive, in part because your kids might decide not to wait. A good approach for a parent who wants to impart both accurate facts and a reminder of their values might sound like this:

> "We have talked about a lot of body-related things. You got more information than I ever had at your age, because I believe that you need that info to keep you safe. I tell you over and over that I will always love you, and that will always be true. Because I love you, I want you to know that I think choosing not to have sex until you're married is really important, too."

Children are going to make great choices, and they're going to screw up—and they might screw up big. When I tell my children there's nothing they can do to make me stop loving them, that is the truth. There is literally nothing. There is also nothing that will shake my unconditional positive regard for my children. I can say this with the confidence I do because I have thought how I would respond to scenarios that range from the most joyous and exciting to the most undesirable, unexpected, or unlikely.

I've thought about what I would say if my child said they're pregnant or their partner was pregnant. How I would thank them for trusting me enough to tell me. How I would remind them that I love them, always. That I would ask, first and foremost, if they felt safe. If their partner was safe. I've thought about how I would educate them on their options and remind them that the decision about what happens next is not mine to make. How I would help them navigate their choices while also respecting my own boundaries. How I might support them in talking to their partner's parents and help them plan for their future, whichever path they chose.

I've reflected on how I would respond if my child came to me and disclosed that they had a STI, knowing that the first step would be to follow up with their usual doctor because they know my child's history and will be able to help set up a course of treatment. I would have to ask the tough questions and see if they know who they might have gotten it from, or if they may have given it to anyone else that needs to be contacted.

I've already had to face a child who told me that they were ready to date. I remember being apprehensive but happy that he had found someone he liked. I wondered if I knew this person, and finding out that I didn't threw me for a loop! I remember feeling like I had to go through every single dating rule and safe-sex tip with him, but talking myself off the ledge and simply reminding my child that he could text me for an out at any point, and that I hoped the person he was going out with was a nice person. Then I sat back to wait for him to get home from his first-ever solo date, and had myself a good ol' thought spiral about what I would do if he came to me and said he was sure he'd met "the one." How it would take Herculean effort to not invalidate his feelings while I tried to steer him back to planning his own future. Turns out, I didn't need to worry about it—he and the lovely young human he went on his first date with broke up after a bit. His next partner was lovely, and they both worked toward lots of different dreams while they were together. Regardless of what happens next, I'm grateful for the thought exercises I've put myself through, just in case he or his sisters ever decide to test me.

Even though I've got one child almost in adulthood, I don't feel like I've got this whole "talking about love, bodies, and sex" thing handled completely, because each and every child is different. The way I address things will need to be tailored to each kid, and I'll need to identify where they need support and where they are ready to fly free. I will have to have conversations with my daughters framed in a different way than I did with my son, because gender impacts the ways people interact with the world, and sex influences the ways we must take care of ourselves.

For example, when it was time to talk to my son about birth control, the options were pretty straightforward because of his biological sex. But if either of my daughters ever come to me asking for birth control, I will have to discuss several different options that vary in suitability based on their intended uses: Are they for controlling cramps? Preventing pregnancy? I will probably have to get in the weeds a bit more than just "there's a box of condoms under the sink, use them if you need them." Unfortunately, for people with a uterus, the systems required to maintain birth control are somewhat more complicated than for people with a penis.

But thankfully I've thought long and hard about how I will carry out these discussions when the time comes. I've reflected on how I will handle each and every one of the above-mentioned scenarios, and several more that I never addressed in this book. And I've made sure that my ideal responses align first and foremost with my beliefs in unconditional positive regard and children's safety. These situations are not easy to think about. I've shed many tears considering what boundaries might look like if I found out my child was actively harming someone. I've calmed my internal rage when I've thought about what it might look like to protect my child if they were being actively hurt. I've researched how to help my child obtain long-term pregnancy protection from methods like implants or shots as a way to keep their future bright and so they would not have to consider any other alternatives. Because I've acknowledged the painful truth that not all sexual encounters are my child's choice. These are hard topics to wrestle with, and I'm so proud of you, reader, for beginning the journey of reflecting on these topics by reading this book.

There is no one-size-fits-all way to have these priceless conversations with our kids, because no two kids are the same. Though I can read through most of this book and repeat the scripts to my children verbatim, you will have to find your voice with your children. You can look through Mechanics and Specifics for inspiration to help guide the talks, but you will find the way to make them the right fit for you and your kids. I know you can do it, because you will have the Foundations of Unconditional Positive Regard, Curiosity, and Consent leading you both through their scary, confusing, hilarious, and unforgettable childhood years. And even if things don't go perfectly—we know they won't—one day you'll wake up to see your functional, happy, adult children, and smile. Because you'll know that you never let the birds, the bees, or the elephant in the room be ignored.

Recommended Resources and Further Reading

General Information and Conversation Starters by Age Range

Early Childhood (birth to age 6)

Books

> *A Little Spot of Emotion Box Set* by Diane Alber (Diane Alber Art LLC, 2020)
>
> *And That's Their Family!* by Kailee Coleman (Kailee Coleman Books, 2021)
>
> *C Is for Consent* by Eleanor Morrison and Faye Orlove (Phonics with Finn, 2018)
>
> *Everyone Poops* by Tarō Gomi (Chronicle Books, 2020)
>
> *The Feelings Book* by Todd Parr (Little, Brown and Company, 2005)
>
> *Look Inside Your Body* by Louie Stowell (Usborne Books, 2014)
>
> *What Makes a Baby* by Cory Silverberg and Fiona Smyth (Triangle Square, 2013)
>
> *Who Has What? All About Girls' Bodies and Boys' Bodies* by Robie H. Harris and Nadine Bernard Westcott (Candlewick, 2011)
>
> *Your Body Belongs to You* by Cornelia Maude Spelman and Teri Weidner (Albert Whitman & Company, 1997)

Middle Childhood (ages 7 to 11)

Books

> *The Boy's Body Book: Everything You Need to Know for Growing Up!*, 5th ed., by Kelli Dunham and Robert Anastas (Applesauce Press, 2019)
>
> *The Care and Keeping of You: The Body Book for Younger Girls*, rev. ed., by Valorie Schaefer and Josee Masse (American Girl Library, 2012)

Consent (for Kids!): Boundaries, Respect, and Being in Charge of YOU by Rachel Brian (Little, Brown Books for Young Readers, 2020)

The Girl's Body Book: Everything Girls Need to Know for Growing Up!, 5th ed., by Kelli Dunham, Laura Tallardy, and Robert Anastas (Applesauce Press, 2019)

Illumanatomy by Kate Davies and Carnovsky (Wide Eyed Editions, 2017)

It's NOT the Stork! A Book About Girls, Boys, Babies, Bodies, Families, and Friends by Robie H. Harris and Michael Emberley (Candlewick, 2008)

My Mind Is a Mountain (Mi mente es una montaña) by Cindy Montenegro and Nqobile Adigun (Lil' Libros, 2022)

Professor Astro Cat's Human Body Odyssey by Dominic Walliman (Flying Eye Books, 2018)

Adolescence (ages 12 to 18)

Books

Are You There, God? It's Me, Margaret., by Judy Blume (Bradbury Press, 1970)

The Care and Keeping of You 2: The Body Book for Older Girls by Cara Natterson and Josee Masse (American Girl Publishing, 2013)

Consent: The New Rules of Sex Education by Jennifer Lang, MD (Althea Press, 2018)

Dating and Sex: A Guide for the 21st Century Teen Boy by Andrew P. Smiler (Margination Press, 2016)

Doing It! by Hannah Witton (Sourcebooks Fire, 2018)

Give Me Some Truth by Eric Gansworth (Arthur A. Levine Books, 2022)

Guy Stuff: The Body Book for Boys by Cara Natterson and Micah Player (American Girl Publishing, 2017)

It's Perfectly Normal: Changing Bodies, Growing Up, Sex, Gender, and Sexual Health by Robie H. Harris and Michael Emberley (Candlewick, 2021)

The Pride Guide: A Guide to Sexual and Social Health for LGBTQ Youth by Jo Langford (Roman & Littlefield, 2018)

The Secret Diary of Adrian Mole, Aged 13¾ by Sue Townsend (HarperTeen, 2003)

S.E.X.: The All-You-Need-to-Know Sexuality Guide to Get You Through Your Teens and Twenties by Heather Corinna (Da Capo Lifelong Books, 2016)

For Caregivers

Books

Forty Fathers: Men Talk about Parenting by Tessa Lloyd (Douglas & McIntyre, 2020)

How to Raise a Boy: The Power of Connection to Build Good Men by Michael C. Reichert (Tarcher Perigee, 2020)

How to Raise a Wild Child by Scott D. Sampson (Mariner, 2016)

Momma Cusses: A Field Guide to Responsive Parenting & Trying Not to Be the Reason Your Kid Needs Therapy by Gwenna Laithland (St. Martin's Essentials, 2024)

The New Puberty: How to Navigate Early Development in Today's Girls by Louise Greenspan, MD, and Julianna Deardorff, PhD (Rodale Books, 2015)

The Power of Showing Up: How Parental Presence Shapes Who Our Kids Become and How Their Brains Get Wired by Daniel J. Siegel, MD, and Tina Payne Bryson, PhD (Ballantine Books, 2021)

Parenting Without Borders: Surprising Lessons Parents Around the World Can Teach Us by Christine Gross-Loy (Avery, 2014)

Raising Boys to be Good Men: A Parent's Guide to Bringing Up Happy Sons in a World Filled with Toxic Masculinity by Aaron Gouveia (Skyhorse Publishing, 2020)

So Sexy So Soon: The New Sexualized Childhood and What Parents Can Do to Protect Their Kids by Diane E. Levin, PhD, and Jean Kilbourne, EdD (Ballantine Books, 2009)

This Is So Awkward: Modern Puberty Explained by Cara Natterson, MD, and Vanessa Kroll Bennett (Rodale Books, 2023)

What Girls Need: How to Raise Bold, Courageous, and Resilient Women by Marisa Porges, PhD (Viking, 2020)

Videos

The Affirmations Song (https://youtu.be/1XYoduQMAjU?si=2G2Q6WVbHkc V0kmX)—A song of positive mantras for children focused on mental health and boundaries.

The Boundary Song (https://youtu.be/aSFvJbSQdA4?si=oItv7To5k5PY7cf0)— Easy, child-friendly song for learning about boundaries.

The Purpose of Friendship (https://youtu.be/aGedUxTAfBk?si=tJ4c_o9xXvZo S1Oq)—Encourages individuals to consider the purpose of their relationships and maintain boundaries on their time and energy.

Tea Consent (https://www.youtube.com/watch?v=oQbei5JGiT8Tea)—An example for caregivers of how to reframe consent in a context apart from sex.

Sexual orientation? Gender identity? What's the difference? (https://youtu.be/C63Xn
--i13o?si=tmigwpTMLIViXCAN)—Concise explanation of identity terms used when discussing LGBTQ+ topics.

Websites, Hotlines, and Resources

AMAZE (amaze.org)—More info. Less weird. Sex education and sexual health information for parents and families.

The Family Acceptance Project (https://familyproject.sfsu.edu/)—San Fransisco State University initiative aiming to promote well-being for LGBTQ+ children and youth through risk prevention.

My Kid Is Gay (mykidisgay.com)—A guide and helpful resources to help parents and families understand their LGBTQ+ kids.

The National Suicide Prevention Lifeline (988lifeline.org)—Provides free and confidential mental health crisis services 24/7 for anyone in distress. Call 988 or 1-800-273-TALK (8255).

PFLAG National (pflag.org)—Dedicated to supporting, educating, and advocating for LGBTQ+ people and their loved ones. Support available at 202-467-8180 and online.

Plan International USA and Promundo, "9 Tips for Parents: Raising Sons to Embrace Healthy, Positive Masculinity" (equimundo.org/wp-content/ uploads 2019/06 healthy-masculinity-tipsheet-for-parents.pdf)—Concrete tips to help parents talk to their sons about healthy masculinity and self-expression, curated by the experts at Plan International USA (an organization for advancing girls' equality and children's rights) and Promundo (a global leader in engaging men and boys in promoting gender equality and preventing violence).

Planned Parenthood for Parents (plannedparenthood.org/learn/parents)— Information to empower parents to have accurate, nonjudgmental conversations with their children about sex, puberty, bodies, and relationships.

RespectAbility (respectability.org)—Sexual education resources that are inclusive of individuals living with intellectual and developmental disabilities.

Scarleteen.com—Billed as "sex-ed for the real world," this site is an inclusive, comprehensive, supportive guide to sexuality and relationships for teens and emerging adults.

SIECUS: Sex Ed for Social Change (siecus.org)—Organization dedicated to advancing comprehensive sex education access through advocacy, policy, and coalition building.

Notes

Chapter 1: Unconditional Positive Regard

17 *recognizing their innate ability to grow and change* Carl R. Rogers, *Client-Centered Therapy: Its Current Practice, Implications, and Theory* (Boston: Houghton Mifflin, 1965).

18 *it also aids in identity development, moral reasoning, and social thinking* B. M. Law, A. M. Siu, and D. T. Shek, "Recognition for Positive Behavior as a Critical Youth Development Construct: Conceptual Bases and Implications on Youth Service Development," *Scientific World Journal* (2012): 809578.

19 *cognitive development occurs over the course of the entire life span* Jean Piaget, "The Theory of Stages in Cognitive Development," in D. R. Green, M. P. Ford, and G. B. Flamer, *Measurement and Piaget* (New York: McGraw-Hill, 1971).

23 *How we as caregivers react* "Positive Parenting Tips," Child Development, Centers for Disease Control and Prevention, last reviewed February 22, 2021, https://www.cdc.gov/ncbddd/childdevelopment/positiveparenting/middle.html.

27 *does not have the positive outcomes we hope for* Nejra Van Zalk, Maria Tillfors, and Kari Trost, "Mothers' and Fathers' Worry and Over-Control: One Step Closer to Understanding Early Adolescent Social Anxiety," *Child Psychiatry & Human Development* 49, no. 6 (2018).

29 *small children are egocentric* Sandra Stojić, Vanja Topić, and Zoltan Nadasdy, "Children and Adults Rely on Different Heuristics for Estimation of Durations," *Scientific Reports* 13, no. 1 (2023), https://doi.org/10.1038/s41598-023-27419-4.

30 *his amygdala had outgrown the rest of his brain* American Academy of Child and Adolescent Psychiatry, "Teen Brain: Behavior, Problem Solving, and Decision Making," *Facts for Families* no. 95 (2017).

32 *developmentally appropriate curiosity* "Normative Sexual Behavior," National Center on the Sexual Behavior of Youth, https://ncsby.org/content/normative-sexual-behavior.

Chapter 2: Curiosity

38 *social learning . . . first studied in children by Albert Bandura in 1961* A. Bandura, D. Ross, and S. A. Ross, "Transmission of Aggression Through Imitation of Aggressive Models," *Journal of Abnormal and Social Psychology* 63, no. 3 (1961).

42 *Curiosity is completely natural, even curiosity about bodies and sex* "Normative Sexual Behavior," National Center on the Sexual Behavior of Youth, https://ncsby.org/content/normative-sexual-behavior.

45 *abstinence-only sex education* K. F. Stanger-Hall and D.W. Hall, "Abstinence-Only Education and Teen Pregnancy Rates: Why We Need Comprehensive Sex Education in the U.S.," *PLoS One* 6, no. 10 (2011): e24658, DOI: 10.1371/journal.pone.0024658.

46 *Providing age-appropriate information makes it measurably more difficult* E. S. Goldfarb and L. D. Lieberman, "Three Decades of Research: The Case for Comprehensive Sex Education," *Journal of Adolescent Health* 68 (2021).

Chapter 3: Consent

57 *the FRIES acronym* "Sexual Consent," Planned Parenthood, n.d., https://plannedparenthood.org/learn/relationships/sexual-consent.

59 *You respect their autonomy* NetSmartzKids, "Who is a 'Trusted Adult'?," National Center for Missing & Exploited Children, n.d., https://www.missingkids.org/content/dam/netsmartz/downloadable/tipsheets/who-is-a-trusted-adult.pdf.

59 *the term "safe adult"* "Child Sexual Abuse Statistics," Rape Abuse and Incest National Network (RAINN), 2015, https://www.rainn.org/articles/child-sexual-abuse.

60 *what qualities make a safe adult* "Safe Adults," Monique Burr Foundation for Children Prevention Education Programs, n.d., https://www.mbfpreventioneducation.org/safe-adults.

62 *Young children . . . should never be asked to keep secrets* Amy Morin, "Talking to Your Kids About Secrets and Privacy," VeryWell Family, updated March 31, 2021, https://www.verywellfamily.com/why-you-shouldnt-tell-your-child-to-keep-secrets-3880039.

63 *believe what they tell you, the first time they tell you* "Step 5: React Responsibly," Darkness to Light, n.d., https://www.d2l.org/education/5-steps/step-5/.

Chapter 5: Self-Stimulation and Exploration

81 *comprehensive, accurate sex education and healthy relationships education is not the norm in the US* "The SIECUS State Profiles," Sex Ed for Social Change, https://siecus.org/state-profiles/.

85 *all examples where concern is warranted* "Warning Signs for Young Children," RAINN, n.d., https://www.rainn.org/articles/warning-signs-young-children.

86 *less likely to be convinced that anyone else should touch them* E. S. Goldfarb,
L. D. Lieberman, "Three Decades of Research: The Case for Comprehensive Sex
Education," *Journal of Adolescent Health* 68 (2021); M. Schneider and J. S. Hirsch,
"Comprehensive Sexuality Education as a Primary Prevention Strategy for Sexual
Violence Perpetration," *Trauma Violence Abuse* 21, no. 3 (July 2020): 439–455,
doi: 10.1177/1524838018772855.

86 *most coexploration between same-age peers* IngBeth Larsson and Carl-
Göran Svedin, "Sexual Experiences in Childhood: Young Adults'
Recollections," *Archives of Sexual Behavior* 31, no. 3 (June 2002):
263–73, DOI:10.1023/a:1015252903931.

86 *not because coexploration with same-age peers is damaging* "Tip Sheet: Age-
Appropriate Sexual Behavior," Stop It Now!, n.d., https://www.stopitnow.org
/ohc-content/age-appropriate-sexual-behavior.

86 *any power imbalance, coercion, threats, or manipulation* "Child Abuse," Mayo Clinic
Child and Family Advocacy Center, n.d., https://www.mayoclinic.org/diseases
-conditions/child-abuse/symptoms-causes/syc-20370864; "Warning Signs for
Young Children," RAINN.

91 *a firmly established sense of privacy that may extend to discussing their bodies* Ross D.
Parke and Douglas B. Sawin, "Children's Privacy in the Home: Developmental,
Ecological, and Child-Rearing Determinants," *Environment and Behavior* 11, no. 1
(1979): 87–104.

92 *Male condoms are one of the most effective and more accessible forms of STI protection
and contraception available* "How effective are condoms?," Planned Parenthood,
n.d., https://www.plannedparenthood.org/learn/birth-control/condom/how
-effective-are-condoms.

94 *Media representations of female pleasure still aren't great* Elizabeth Letsou, "Why the
Proper Representation of Female Pleasure on Television Matters," Her Campus,
March 1, 2021, https://www.hercampus.com/culture/female-pleasure
-representation-television/.

Chapter 6: Periods, Period.

105 *Treating menstruation this way . . . can help prevent children from developing feelings of fear and shame* M. C. McHugh, "Menstrual Shame: Exploring
the Role of 'Menstrual Moaning,'" in C. Bobel, I .T. Winkler, B. Fahs, et al.,
The Palgrave Handbook of Critical Menstruation Studies (Singapore: Palgrave
MacMillan, 2020), https://www.ncbi.nlm.nih.gov/books/NBK565666/
doi: 10.1007/978-981-15-0614-7_32.

106 *Your vagina does not need soap or water or anything else in it to keep it clean*
Andrea Eisenberg, "Your Vagina is Self Cleaning," Michican Women's Health,
September 22, 2021, http://michiganwomensobgyn.com/your-vagina-is-self
-cleaning/.

109 *as early as age eight or nine, but generally speaking around age eleven or twelve* Gladys M. Martinez, "Trends and Patterns in Menarche in the United States: 1995 through 2013-2017" *National Health Statistics Reports,* 146 (2020).

111 *there is some evidence that the aluminum isn't good for us* P. D. Darbre, "Aluminium, Antiperspirants and Breast Cancer," *Journal of Inorganic Biochemistry* 99, no. 9 (2005): 1912–19.

Chapter 7: Pen15 Club

134 *Shampoo, conditioner, and soap can all irritate your urethra and give you an infection* "5 Reasons Not to Masturbate with Soap," Condomania, December 27, 2021, https://condomania.com/a/blog/5-reasons-not-to-masturbate-with-soap.

135 *scientific results that tell us this binary is patently false* Y. J. Wong and A. B. Rochlen, "Demystifying Men's Emotional Behavior: New Direction and Implications for Counseling and Research," *Psychology of Men & Masculinity* 6, no. 1 (2005): 62–72, https://doi.org/10.1037/1524-9220.6.1.62.

Chapter 8: Where Do Babies Come From?

142 *a theory called scaffolding* L. S. Vygotsky, "Interaction Between Learning and Development," in M. Cole, V. John-Steiner, S. Scribner, and E. Souberman, eds., *Mind in Society* (Cambridge, MA: Harvard University Press, 1935/1978), 79–91.

143 *theory posits that children do not develop the ability to see other people's perspectives* H. Wimmer and H. Mayringer, "False Belief Understanding in Young Children: Explanations Do Not Develop Before Predictions," *International Journal of Behavioral Development* 22 no. 2 (1998): 403–22, https://doi.org/10.1080/016502598384441.

148 *what those in psychology refer to as schema* American Psychological Association, "Schema," APA Dictionary of Psychology, https://dictionary.apa.org/schema.

Chapter 9: The Feels

167 *intimacy is the bond one individual forms with another (or others)* G. M. Timmerman, "A Concept Analysis of Intimacy," *Issues in Mental Health Nursing* 12, no. 1 (1991): 19–30, DOI: 10.3109/01612849109058207.

167 *intimacy can generally be broken down into four different types: emotional, mental, spiritual, and physical* Carmen Cuisido, "How to Nourish Different Types of Intimacy in Your Relationship," Psych Central, August 18, 2022, https://psychcentral.com/relationships/nourishing-the-different-types-of-intimacy-in-your-relationship.

169 *Robert Sternberg proposed what he called the triangular theory of love* R. J. Sternberg, "A Triangular Theory of Love," *Psychological Review* 93 (1986): 119–35.

180 *most teens in the US wait until seventeen to have sex* "United States Teens," Guttmacher Institute, accessed November 8, 2023, http://www.guttmacher.org/united-states/teens; "Youth Risk Behavior Survey Data Summary & Trends

Report," Centers for Disease Control and Prevention, 2011–2021, https://www.cdc.gov/healthyyouth/data/yrbs/pdf/YRBS_Data-Summary-Trends_Report2023_508.pdf.

Chapter 10: Consent NOW

194 *hormones are responsible for a myriad of changes, and also for a potential increase in sexual curiosity and the beginnings of sexual attraction* "Normative Sexual Behavior," National Center on the Sexual Behavior of Youth, https://ncsby.org/content/normative-sexual-behavior; J. Dennis Fortenbery, "Puberty and Adolescent Sexuality," *Hormones and Behavior* 64, no. 2 (2013): 280–87.

Chapter 11: The Five Pillars of Safe Sex

215 *a lot of people would benefit from including lubrication in their sex lives* Caitlin E. Kennedy, Ping Teresa Yeh, Jingjia Li, Lianne Gonsalves, and Manjulaa Narasimhan, "Lubricants for the Promotion of Sexual Health and Well-Being: A Systematic Review," *Sexual and Reproductive Health Matters* 29, no. 3 (2022): 2044198, DOI: 10.1080/26410397.2022.2044198.

222 *anal sex should always involve additional lubrication* "Butt What About Lube?," Ending HIV, September 12, 2023, http://www.endinghiv.org/au/blog/butt-what-about-lube.

223 *no way during sex to tell if the other person has orgasmed unless you ask* "Can a man tell if a woman orgasms?," Go Ask Alice!, Columbia University, updated September 11, 2020, https://goaskalice.columbia.edu/answered-questions/how-to-tell-if-woman-orgasms.

Chapter 13: "The Internet Is for Porn" —*Avenue Q*

247 *age of first exposure to pornography has gotten younger* "Age and Experience of First Exposure to Pornography: Relations to Masculine Norms," Poster Session, Thursday, August 3, 11–11:50 a.m. EDT, Halls D and E, Level 2, Walter E. Washington Convention Center, 801 Mount Vernon Pl NW, Washington, DC; Michael B. Robb and Supreet Mann, "Teens and Pornography," Common Sense Media, January 10, 2023, https://www.commonsensemedia.org/sites/default/files/research/report/2022-teens-and-pornography-final-web.pdf; S. Astle, N. Leonhardt, and B. Willoughby, "Home Base: Family of Origin Factors and the Debut of Vaginal Sex, Anal Sex, Oral Sex, Maturbation, and Pornography Use in a National Sample of Adolescents," *Journal of Sex Research* 57 (2020): 1089–99, https://doi.org/10.1080/00224499.2019.1691140.

248 *evidence that sexualized human bodies have been a point of curiosity for human beings for centuries* Philip S. Rawson, *Erotic Art of the East: The Sexual Theme in Oriental*

Painting and Sculpture (New York: Putnam, 1968), 380; John R. Clark, *Roman Sex: 100 B.C. to A.D. 250* (New York: Harry N. Abrams, 2003), 168.

259 *rate of porn addiction in young people* "Pornography Use Among Teen Statistics," Youth Pornography Addiction Center, accessed November 8, 2023, https://www.ypacenter.com/youth-pornography-addiction.

Chapter 14: Pride

264 *discuss some definitions and clarify some concepts* "Sexual Orientation and Gender Identity Definitions," Human Rights Campaign, HRC Foundation, accessed November 8, 2023, https://www.hrc.org/resources/sexual-orientation-and-gender-identity-terminology-and-definitions.

266 *lesbian, gay, and bisexual children who were rejected by their families were 8.4 times more likely to have attempted suicide* Caitlin Ryan, David Huebner, Rafael M. Diaz, and Jorge Sanchez, "Family Rejection as a Predictor of Negative Health Outcomes in White and Latino Lesbian, Gay, and Bisexual Young Adults," *Pediatrics* 123, no. 1 (2009): 346–52, DOI: 10.1542/peds.2007-3524.

266 *Family acceptance has been found to be a protective factor for LGBTQ+ youth* Caitlin Ryan, Stephen T. Russell, David Huebner, Rafael Diaz, and Jorge Sanchez, "Family Acceptance in Adolescence and the Health of LGBT Young Adults," *Journal of Child and Adolescent Psychiatric Nursing* 23, no. 4 (2010): 205–13.

267 *LGBTQ+ youth who are bullied at school about their identity* Valerie A. Earnshaw, Laura M. Bogart, V. Paul Poteat, Sari L. Reisner, and Mark A. Schuster, "Bullying Among Lesbian, Gay, Bisexual, and Transgender Youth," *Pediatric Clinics of North America* 63, no. 6 (2016): 999–1010, https://doi.org/10.1016/j.pcl.2016.07.004.

267 *Cultural ideas like slang, rules and norms, and how to navigate the social aspects of their identity* Joanne R. Smith, "Group Norms," Oxford Research Encyclopedias, May 29, 2020, https://doi.org/10.1093/acrefore/9780190236557.013.453.

271 *the survey of US census information from 2021* "Household Pulse Survey," US Census Bureau, July 21–September 13, 2021, https://www.census.gov/library/stories/2021/11/census-bureau-survey-explores-sexual-orientation-and-gender-identity.html.

276 *choosing to use alternative, agreed-upon names for certain body parts may be a way to ease communication and improve discomfort* Anouk Verveen, Baudewijntje P. C. Kreukels, Nastasja M. de Graaf, and Thomas D Steensma, "Body Image in Children with Gender Incongruence," *Clinical Child Psychology and Psychiatry* 23, no. 3 (2021): 839–54, DOI: 10.1177.13591045211000797.

Acknowledgments

First and foremost, this book would not have been possible without my children. Thank you for being my inspirations, my guinea pigs, my successes, my spirit lifters, my motivation, my Peanut Butter, my Turkey Toes, and my Googums. Thank you for putting up with Mama spending long days on the computer, and thank you for always knowing just when to distract me. WoahWoah, thank you for watching your sisters and telling me when I'm full of crap. YaYa, thank you for giving me snuggles and always being willing to help. VV, thank you for helping me learn to laugh again, and for (sometimes) being willing to compromise. I love you and I'm so proud of all of you.

Next, I need to try to figure out exactly how to thank my sister. I'm not exactly sure it's possible, but I'll give it a try. Dori: Without your practical support (so many meals, trips to the Dark Orca, and kid-wrangling), intellectual support (way to go, Spock), and emotional support (I promise to stop FaceTiming you *quite* so often, unless I'm in Target), I would not have been able to power through the writing and revising of this manuscript. Heck, let's be honest—I'm not sure I would have been able to power through this much of adulthood without you. I'm so glad you're my best-friend-sister.

Thank you to WilT for providing so much practical support—babysitting, home construction, garbage disposal, and demolition. You are a really cool human who is going to do cool, potentially scary stuff with your life. I love you and I'm proud of you, too.

Thank you to Philip for allowing me to use our childhood as a guide and for all the snuggles with the kids—I owe you a Spirit Jersey.

Thank you, Ben, for definitely NOT giving me legal advice, for being part of my childhood shenanigans, for listening to book ramblings, and for spoiling my kids.

Kayla, thank you for the laughs, the niblings, the Disney, and the kindred spirit bonus family. SISTER TRIP?!

Thank you to Marissa and Mauri for the GIANT BRAINS you lent me, along with the excellent advice and timely academic resources. I admire your knowledge, and I'm so grateful that we're friends and colleagues because hot diggity, did y'all make this book better. Plus, you make my life better, so thanks for that, too.

To my amazing agent, Amy Collins—thank you for taking a chance on me and for being such a fierce advocate. I would never have made it this far without such a competent, compassionate, knowledgeable person at the helm. I'm so excited for the next one (after I get a LOT of sleep).

Thank you, Jessica, for your patience, guidance, and expertise in the publishing world. I don't imagine that everyone gets an amazing editor right out of the gate, and I am so grateful I did.

Juliana, thank you for facilitating all things, coordinating all things, saving my bacon, and having a super-kick-butt favorite animal.

Grandma Peg, thank you for helping to keep my home livable as I navigate the ever-changing landscape of my life. I'm so lucky that we can call you family.

To B'Wanda, AhMee, Erin, Kim, Bess, Pritt, Beckles, Lisa, Josi, Jenna, and Ben-With-The-No-Hair—thank you for being listening ears, providers of feedback, fonts of wisdom, carers of children, beacons of clarity, and just all-around amazing humans. I wouldn't be where I am today without each of you in my life.

To Gwenna, Tori, and Emily—thank you for always being in my pocket, and in my corner. You have taught me so much about what we do, and how to do it well. You push me to be better and push back when I'm getting too big for my britches. Plus, y'all are hilarious.

Abbi, thank you for being a brave, thoughtful, funny, wise kid. I'm honored you let me include some of your thoughts and experiences in this manuscript.

To the folks who agreed to let me share some of their stories—thank you for allowing me to include you in this book. With any luck, your stories will go on to help parents across the country (and maybe even the world!) navigate the choppy waters of sex ed with their kids. You are all heroes in my eyes.

To my mom—even when my going got tough and I made some . . . interesting . . . decisions, you never strayed from being my supporter. I owe a great deal of my perspective as a parent to you, and I feel so lucky that my kids have you as a Nana. I love you.

To my dad—143. Forever.

To Jimb—I can't believe I did it. I would say I hope you're proud of me, but I'm lucky enough to know that you are. Love you > ∞

Index

C

child development theories, 17, 142–43, 153. *See also* cognitive development; *specific topics*

childhood. *See* adolescence; early childhood; *specific topics*

children. *See* child development theories; consent; specific topics

cloth pads, for periods, 114

coercion, 199–200, 208, 280

cognitive development
abstract thought development as part of, 20, 34, 54
concrete operational stage of, 20
formal operational stage of, 20, 194
Piaget's theory of, 19–21
preoperational stage of, 20, 76–77
sensorimotor stage of, 19
theory of mind, 143

communication, 174, 203–4, 213–14, 219–21, 226

compatibility, in relationships, 177–78

condoms, use of, 92, 139, 202–3

consent, children and, 12, 15. *See also* body autonomy
boundary phrases, 64
communication as element of, 203–4
dating and, 196
enthusiastic participation and, 216–17, 222–25, 226
in Five Pillars of Safe Sex, 213
FRIES acronym, 57–59, 191–92, 206–7
giving/revoking practices for, 64
health issues and, 55, 64
impaired, 208
language for, 53–54
legal age of, 208
modeling of, 64
physical, 68
safe adults and, 59–64, 76

safety issues and, 55–56, 64
tacit permission myth and, 197–98
variabilities in communication style for, 56

Consent for Knowledge, 12, 67, 69–79, 163, 268

consequences, 23, 25–26, 28–29

curiosity, self-esteem and, 257–58. *See also specific topics*

D

dating, conversations about
during adolescence, 196–97, 235–41
age-setting for, 231, 233–35
boundary-setting and, 236–38
coercion and, 199–200, 208
condoms and, 202–3
consent and, 196
definition of, 230
mistakes during, 239–41
Number Twelve Rule, 194–95, 231–35
opting out of, 241–43
peer pressure and, 196–97, 200
in popular culture, 230–31
rape and, 198–99
readiness for, 195
tacit permission myth, 197–98

decision-making, self-awareness and, 170–75

disposable pads, for periods, 114

"don't" statements, 24–25

dress and appearance, 182–85

E

early childhood, conversations during, 107, 131, 152–56

emotions, expression of, 111–12, 135–38

erections, 123–33, 139

exploration. *See* bodily exploration; sexual exploration

mistakes, 23, 25–26, 31, 34, 239–41, 260–61
morality, about sexual behaviors, 140–41
moral reasoning, 18

N
NEMOURS KidsHealth, 47
nocturnal emissions, 130
Number Twelve Rule, about dating, 194–95, 231–35

O
orgasm, 96, 134, 223

P
parents, parenting approaches and, 11, 14–15, 24–25, 48–51, 59–60, 99–100. *See also* safe adults
penis, 36, 43, 77, 93–95, 139, 151, 274. *See also* erections; reproduction
Period Preparedness Packs, 110
periods. *See* menstruation
period underwear, 115
Piaget, Jean, 19–21, 143, 194. *See also* cognitive development
Pink Tax, 113
Planned Parenthood, FRIES acronym, 57–59
"playing doctor," 31–33
polycystic ovarian syndrome, 121
pornography
 adolescent exposure to, 249–54
 age of exposure to, 247–48
 curiosity about, 249–50, 254–55, 262
 as false representation of real sexual behaviors, 251–52, 262
 Five Pillars of Safe Sex, 253
 grooming and, 255–56
 history of, 248

mistakes over, 260–61
 safety and, 254–55
pregnancy, conversations about, 141–42, 146–50, 155–60
preschool children, sexual exploration conversations with, 88
primary caregivers, 18. *See also* parents
puberty, 30, 46, 109–12. *See also* adolescence; menstruation

Q
queer relationships, 277

R
rape, as sexual violence, 71, 198–99, 208
relationships, conversations about, 166–70, 172–79, 187–88. *See also* dating; intimacy
reproduction, reproductive systems and, conversations about. *See also* penis; pregnancy; vagina
 during adolescence, 157
 biological processes of, 144–45, 151–52, 161
 birth processes, 148–50
 cell division in, 150–52
 for early to middle childhood, 152–56
 magical thinking about, 158–59
respect, 33, 174
responsibility, in relationships, 176
Rogers, Carl, 17
Ross, Bob, 14, 73–74
rules, boundary-setting and, 27, 44

S
safe adults, 59, 60–64, 76, 153
safe sex. *See* Five Pillars of Safe Sex
safety, 55–56, 64, 174–75, 254–55. *See also* safe adults
scaffolding, 142–43, 153

About the Author

Rachel Coler Mulholland is a counselor and university professor from small-town Minnesota. She has dual bachelor's degrees in psychology and human services, and a master's degree in clinical mental health counseling. While living in rural Minnesota, Rachel has provided mental health skills training for children with severe emotional disturbance in a school-based day treatment program, school-based counseling for high school students, and counseling for college students of varying ages. She focuses her course objectives and professional energy on resilience development, trauma-informed therapeutic interventions, assertive communication, interpersonal skills, and self-efficacy.

In addition to her academic work, Rachel spends a little bit of her free time traveling, doing home renovations, and making parenting content on social media. The bulk of her free time is spent doing fun stuff with her three kids, like driving them to dance or theater, watching their sporting events, and getting her butt kicked at video games. She also enjoys karaoke, an ever-changing array of crafty hobbies, and almost winning at trivia.